Sleep Well Tonight!

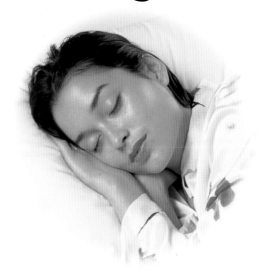

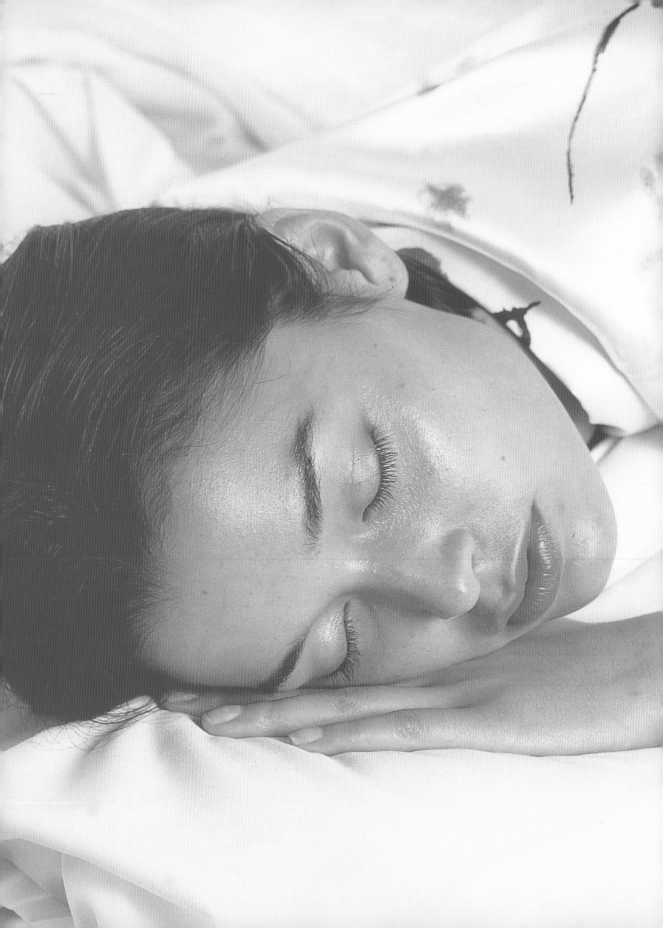

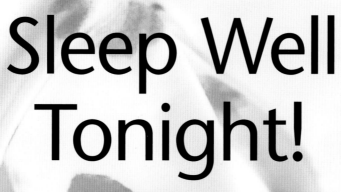

Sleep Well Tonight!

Sure-fire solutions for a good night's rest

Harriet Griffey

Sterling Publishing Co., Inc.
New York
A Sterling/Silver Book

A QUARTO BOOK

Library of Congress Cataloging-in-Publication Data is available upon request.

Published by
Sterling Publishing Co., Inc
387 Park Avenue South
New York, NY 10016-8810

This book was designed and produced by
Quarto Publishing plc
The Old Brewery
6 Blundell Street
London N7 6BH

Senior editor **Michelle Pickering**
Editor **Mary Senechal**
Senior art editor **Penny Cobb**
Designer **Simon Wilder**
Illustrator **Stuart Robertson/ The Ink Shed**
Photographer **Richard Gleed, Paul Forrester**
Art director **Moira Clinch**

Typeset by Central Southern Typesetters, Eastbourne, UK
Manufactured by Regent Publishing Services Ltd, Hong Kong
Printed by Leefung-Asco Printers Ltd, China

ISBN 0-8069-6313-1

NOTE
This book is not intended as a substitute for the advice of a health care professional, particularly with respect to symptoms that may require diagnosis or medical attention.

C O N

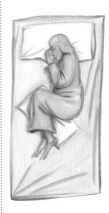

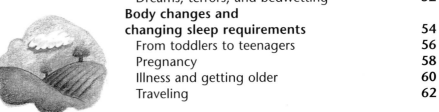

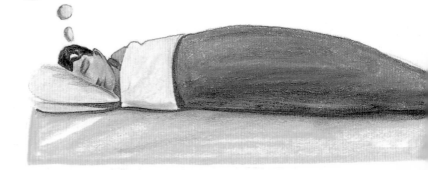

T E N T S

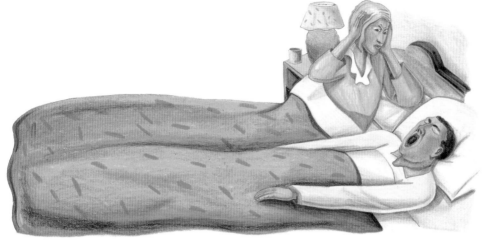

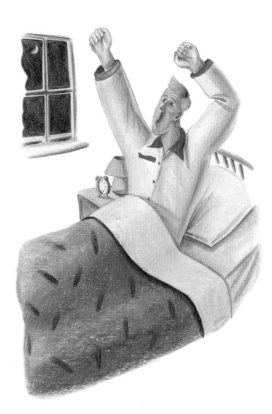

Introduction

Sleep that knits up the ravell'd sleeve of care,

The depth of each day's life, sore labour's bath,

Balm of hurt minds, great nature's second course,

Chief nourisher in life's feast.

Macbeth (act II, scene ii)

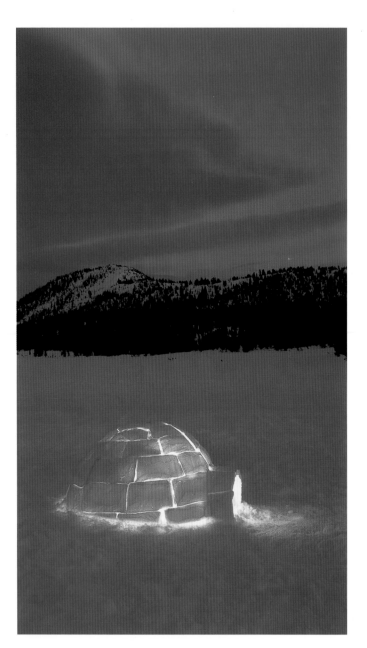

◄ *People who have to adapt to shorter daylight hours, such as the Eskimos of the Arctic Circle, often do so by sleeping more.*

Sleep is perhaps the most mysterious of all our natural body functions. Some of us sleep heavily, some of us sleep lightly, and some people sleep hardly at all. Patterns of sleep are almost as individual as the world's population itself. We know that sleep waves and dreaming (or REM) phases occur – but there is little real knowledge of why, and what their importance might be. Even the experts agree that sleep studies are in their infancy. We can measure the effects of lack of sleep more easily than its benefits, and make deductions from that, but fundamentally all we know is that the best cure for sleepiness is sleep itself.

Twenty-five years sleep

We spend around one third of our lives asleep, which could mount up to 25 years or more. That is provided we sleep the optimum 8 hours out of every 24. Some people are renowned for sleeping much less than that, partly, it is said, to benefit from the additional time available for activity when they reduce the hours of sleep.

Salvador Dali apparently so resented spending time asleep that he switched to dozing. He would hold a teaspoon in his hand, balanced over a tin plate, so that the moment he drifted off and let go of the spoon, the noise woke him. Perhaps this explains the surreal, dreamlike quality of his paintings. Leonardo da Vinci was said to sleep for only an hour and a half each day, in a series

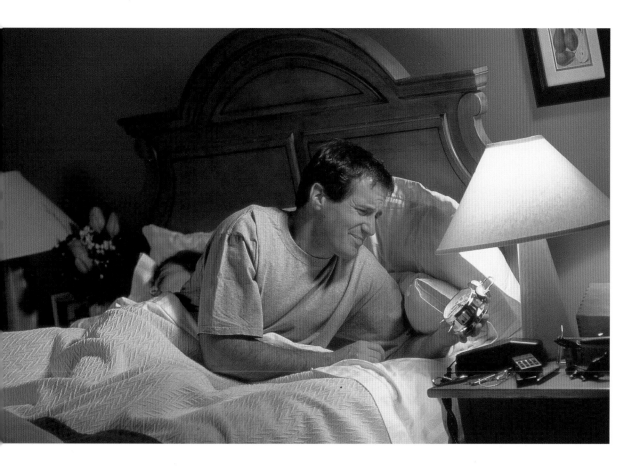

of 15-minute naps, which may help to explain his phenomenal output. This habit of napping is known to sleep researchers as polyphasic ultra-short sleep.

▲ Sleep can sometimes prove elusive, and knowing how to handle periods of sleeplessness can be beneficial.

Unusual sleep habits

Margaret Thatcher, Mussolini, Hitler, and Mao Tse-tung are just some examples of the 5 percent of people who can happily exist on only three or four hours sleep a night. Well-known afternoon-nappers include Winston Churchill and Johannes Brahms, who is reputed to have dozed off while composing his famous Lullaby. Eskimos, who endure the long winter nights of the Arctic Circle without artificial light, adapt by sleeping an extra four hours a night. An Italian scientist who spent nine months isolated in an underground chamber –

◄ Peaceful sleep is essential for health and well-being, as it is during sleep that the body's restorative functions take place.

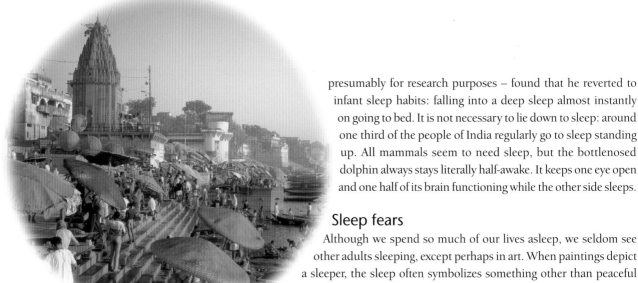

presumably for research purposes – found that he reverted to infant sleep habits: falling into a deep sleep almost instantly on going to bed. It is not necessary to lie down to sleep: around one third of the people of India regularly go to sleep standing up. All mammals seem to need sleep, but the bottlenosed dolphin always stays literally half-awake. It keeps one eye open and one half of its brain functioning while the other side sleeps.

Sleep fears

Although we spend so much of our lives asleep, we seldom see other adults sleeping, except perhaps in art. When paintings depict a sleeper, the sleep often symbolizes something other than peaceful slumber. Sleep can represent vulnerability, or human weakness, or laziness and sloth. And sleep is often a metaphor for death. People talk in euphemistic terms about putting a beloved pet "to sleep," or tell a child that someone who died "fell asleep and didn't wake up." We also hear of people dying in their sleep. All of this can make us fear sleep. And even the prospect of dreaming – when we rehearse some of our deepest fears – can be frightening.

That sleep is sometimes elusive, or even impossible, should come as no surprise. We live complex and busy lives that are occasionally stressful; and we are responsive

▲ *Around a third of the population of India regularly sleep standing up.*

▼ *Dolphins never completely sleep; part of their brain always remains alert.*

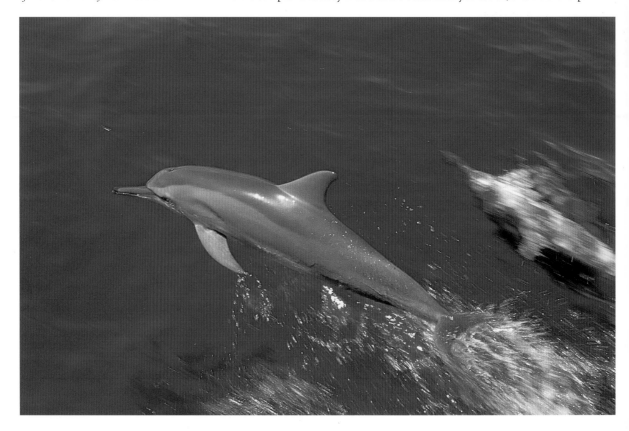

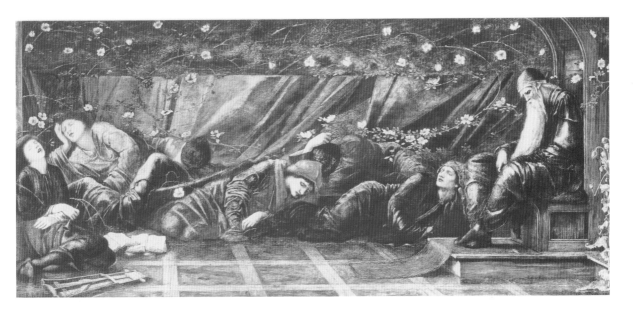

to all manner of outside influences and psychological promptings that can keep us tense and alert. The key is to acknowledge how your daily life can affect your ability to sleep, and to believe that you can achieve peaceful sleep once more. By understanding the information that we do have about sleep and individual sleep needs, you can reduce the anxiety that arises during periods when sleep is difficult to come by.

▲ *The mythology of the sleeping beauty has captured many people's imaginations, including Edward Burne Jones in his* Briar Rose *series of paintings.*

Sleep management

This can't always be done overnight, and can require some thought and application. The purpose of this book is two-fold: to provide an immediate course of action, the Crisis Management Plan, to begin the process; and additional resources for addressing your sleeping patterns and needs on a more lasting basis. For many, the Crisis Management Plan will solve a short-term problem, and its practice may even reduce the possibility of a relapse. Understanding why the difficulty occurred in the first place, and knowing what self-help measures to take can only be beneficial. The Sleep Education section will help you to understand your sleep problem, and Sleep Solutions outlines a range of natural therapies useful for tackling such problems. Making changes now could mean a major improvement in your general health, and never having to suffer a sleep problem again.

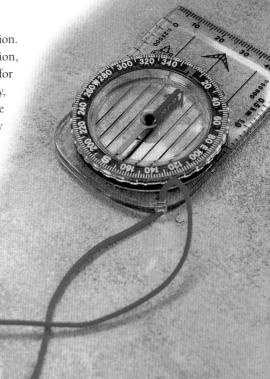

▶ *There are many natural approaches that can help to solve sleep problems. Feng shui, for example, gives guidance on the best direction in which to sleep.*

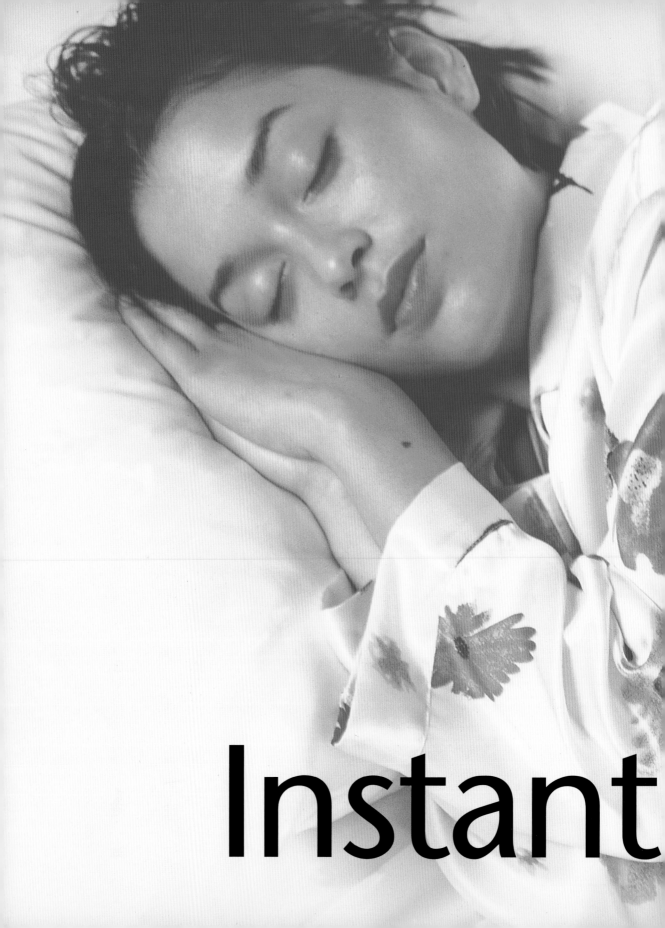

Instant

Whatever your sleep problem, you can take steps today to improve the quality and the quantity of your sleep. Introducing effective sleep patterns means exploring the reasons for your problem, and the Crisis Management Plan outlined in the following pages begins that process. Taking those first steps, and feeling confident of their effectiveness, as you learn more about the function of sleep and how to meet your individual needs, is the key to solving both short- and long-term problems.

Solutions

Crisis Management Plan

By following the plan below, you can begin to increase the likelihood of sleeping well. You could sleep better on the first night of this plan, but think in terms of a progressive improvement over an initial period of seven nights. That way, you can be more relaxed about solving your problem, which is helpful in itself.

What to Do Today

Although you don't plan to sleep until after you go to bed tonight, what you do during today will influence your ability both to go to sleep and stay asleep.

1

Do get up at a reasonable hour.

Do set your alarm if necessary, and make sure you get out of bed when it rings.

Don't be tempted to rest in the morning to compensate for a bad night's sleep or for going to bed late the night before.

Do get up earlier, and you will be able to sleep earlier: being unable to fall asleep when you go to bed and waking up late are linked.

2 **Don't** be tempted to sleep or catnap during the day. Any daytime sleep detracts from your ability to fall asleep, and stay sleeping peacefully, at night. If you feel like napping during the day, take a walk instead.

3 **Do** make sure you get some exercise today, and preferably some fresh air – walking can usefully combine both. If you work out, or do any form of vigorous activity, have your session in the earlier part of the day. Energetic exercise late at night over-stimulates the body, raising the temperature and metabolic rate (the rate at which continuous bodily processes occur). Making love is the only physical exercise recommended immediately before sleep: it can increase the body's production of endorphins – pain-relieving substances – and other chemicals that enhance relaxation and sleepiness.

4 **Do** eat regularly. Have three well-balanced meals, the largest for lunch and the last at least two hours before you go to bed. A light snack, perhaps with a milky drink, about an hour before bed can also help.

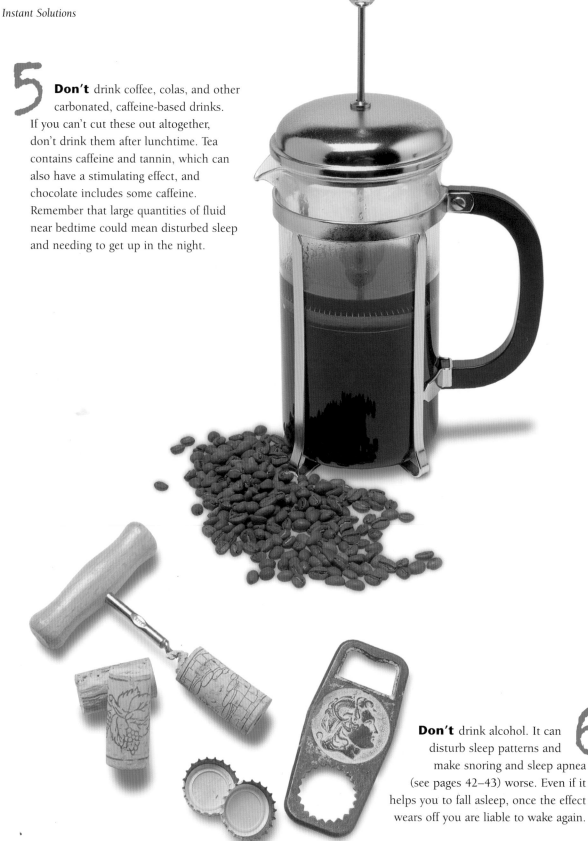

5 **Don't** drink coffee, colas, and other carbonated, caffeine-based drinks. If you can't cut these out altogether, don't drink them after lunchtime. Tea contains caffeine and tannin, which can also have a stimulating effect, and chocolate includes some caffeine. Remember that large quantities of fluid near bedtime could mean disturbed sleep and needing to get up in the night.

6 **Don't** drink alcohol. It can disturb sleep patterns and make snoring and sleep apnea (see pages 42–43) worse. Even if it helps you to fall asleep, once the effect wears off you are liable to wake again.

7 **Don't** smoke: the nicotine in cigarettes is a stimulant. Smoking and its side-effects – which include catarrh, coughing, and blocked sinuses – all contribute to poor sleep patterns.

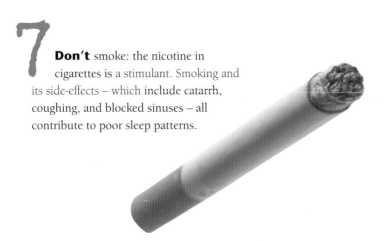

8 **Don't** keep thinking about how tired you are, and how anxious you are feeling about a sleep problem. Although this is difficult, resist the temptation and find some displacement activity, such as reading, listening to music, or taking a walk.

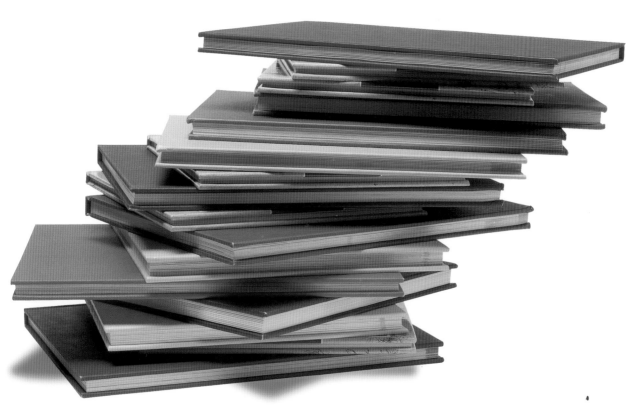

What to Do When You Go to Bed

Your bedtime routine should help you begin to prepare for sleep. Allow time for this part of the relaxation process. Very few people can work all-out until late at night, throw themselves into bed, and sleep peacefully. Most of us need an easing-off period that enables the body and mind to adjust to the inevitability of sleep.

Do make sure that your bedroom is a peaceful, inviting place to be, uncluttered, and without a television or telephone.

Do make sure your bedroom is comfortably warm when you go to bed, and well-ventilated. The recommended temperature is around 65°F (18°C). If the atmosphere is dry or stuffy, increase the humidity by using a vaporizer, placing bowls of water in the room, or draping damp towels over the radiator.

16

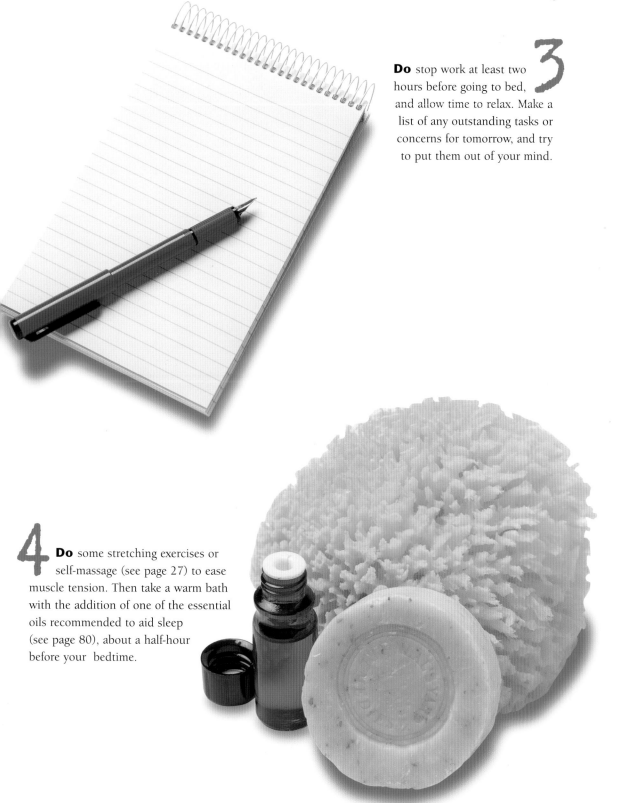

Do stop work at least two 3
hours before going to bed,
and allow time to relax. Make a
list of any outstanding tasks or
concerns for tomorrow, and try
to put them out of your mind.

4 **Do** some stretching exercises or
self-massage (see page 27) to ease
muscle tension. Then take a warm bath
with the addition of one of the essential
oils recommended to aid sleep
(see page 80), about a half-hour
before your bedtime.

5 **Do** switch off the phone, or put on the answerphone; a conversation will disrupt your bedtime routine.

6 **Don't** go to bed too early; only go to bed prior to sleep. Read a book or listen to some relaxing music as you settle down. Allow some time to feel drowsy before turning out the light to sleep.

7 **Do** have a milky drink, a chamomile tea, or a herbal infusion or decoction known to aid sleep (see pages 102–103).

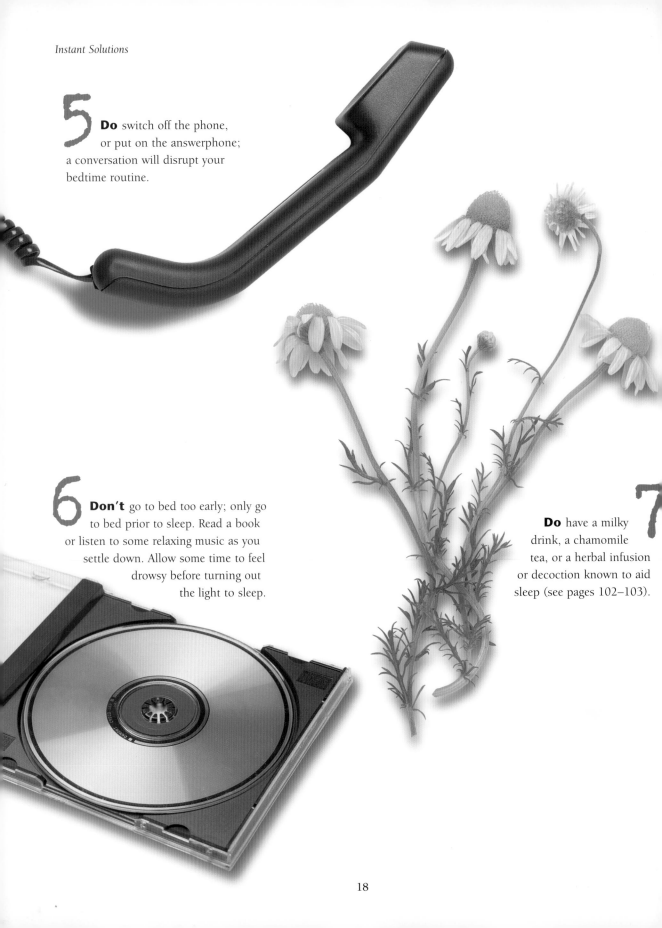

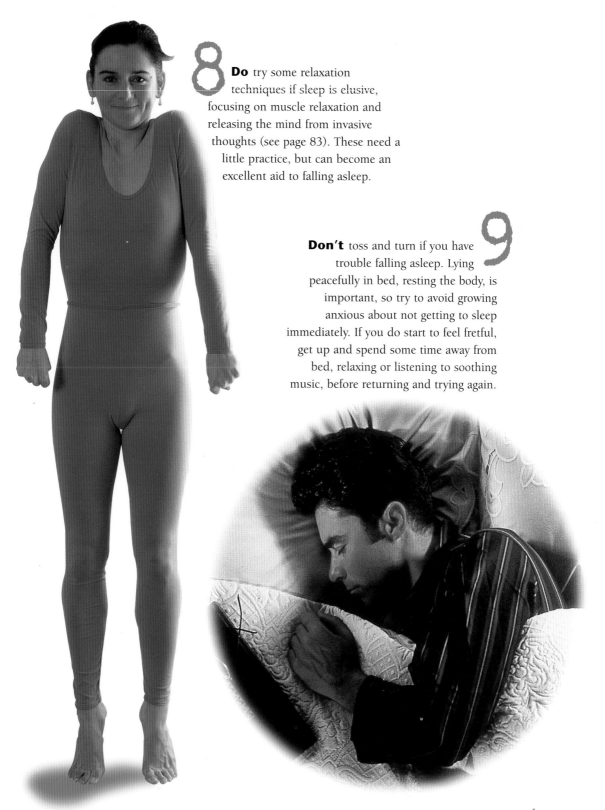

8 Do try some relaxation techniques if sleep is elusive, focusing on muscle relaxation and releasing the mind from invasive thoughts (see page 83). These need a little practice, but can become an excellent aid to falling asleep.

9 Don't toss and turn if you have trouble falling asleep. Lying peacefully in bed, resting the body, is important, so try to avoid growing anxious about not getting to sleep immediately. If you do start to feel fretful, get up and spend some time away from bed, relaxing or listening to soothing music, before returning and trying again.

19

Sleep Hygiene

Sleep hygiene is a term used by professionals to describe the general and practical advice that can promote good sleep patterns. Sleep hygiene is also concerned with what you do prior to attempting sleep.

▶ *The exhaustion of early parenthood is caused, almost exclusively, by the unsettled sleep habits of a new baby*

▼ *The stress caused by excessive pressures of work can extend beyond the confines of the waking day and lead to disrupted sleep.*

The principles of sleep hygiene influence the recommendations made in the Crisis Management Plan, but a more detailed understanding helps you to diagnose why sleep is elusive, and how bad your sleep problem is. Reestablishing a good sleep pattern may take several weeks if it is preceded by long-term irregularities. If there is no improvement after all self-help measures have been taken, it is important to discover and treat whatever underlying problem is involved. However, consulting a doctor before taking self-help steps may be counterproductive, as most doctors will recommend such measures before any further assessment and diagnosis.

Sleep is so integral to our lives that a consistent deficit can make a big difference to how we feel and manage day to day. Consequently, it is important to redress sleep problems

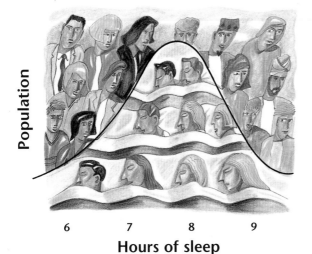

Population / **Hours of sleep**

6   7   8   9

▲ *Most people function best on a regular seven- to eight-hour sleep pattern, although some people need more sleep than this and some can manage on considerably less.*

when they arise. Around one third of us suffer from sleep problems at some time, and women are twice as likely to have their sleep affected than men.

The three main areas of sleep hygiene are the sleeping environment, exercise, and diet. Many of us fall into bad habits without realizing it. Pressures of work can mean burning the midnight oil and depending on sleep to keep the balance, when a period of relaxation is also necessary. For the parents of small children, endless night wakings can induce poor sleep periods. A reevaluation is necessary and implementing change becomes essential.

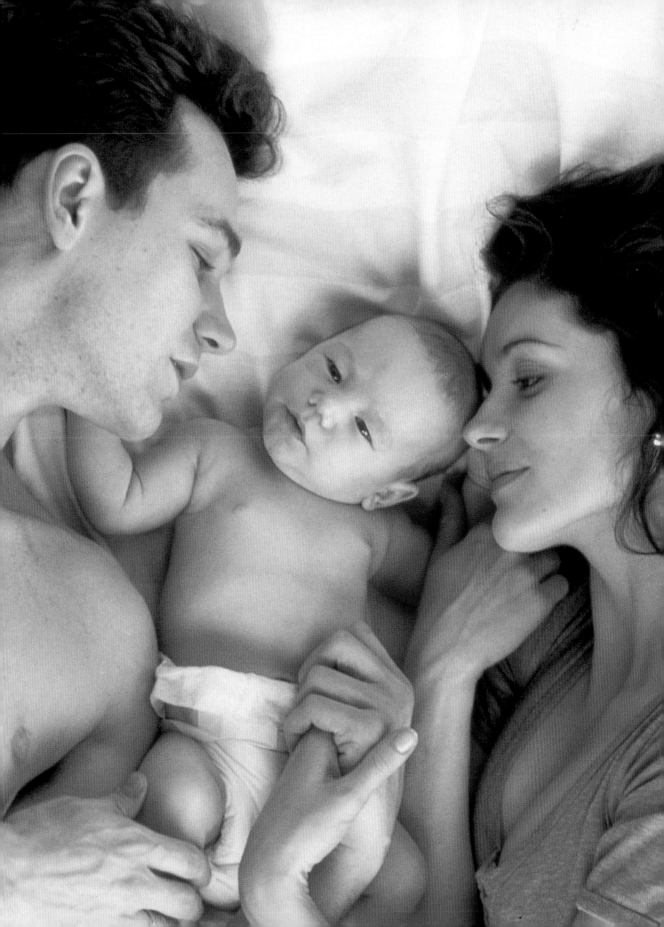

Where You Sleep

We spend around one third of our lives sleeping, or trying to, so the environment in which we sleep – the bedroom – should be specifically geared to the purpose. Ideally, a bedroom should be associated solely with going to sleep – if it must double as a study or living room, its primary focus should be sleeping.

The Bed

The most important item in the bedroom is the bed. Is it big enough? Is it too soft, so that you wake every morning with a crick in your neck? Is it so hard that you start the day with a sore hip-bone? Do you spend half the night trying to squirm out of the dip in the middle? Any such factors will disturb your sleep, as you desperately try to get comfortable during the night.

Ideally your bed should include a mattress with springs which doesn't sag; turning the mattress regularly can help avoid this. It should be firm enough to support the back, especially as during "paradoxical" sleep – also known as REM or dreaming sleep – (see pages 34–35), when the body's muscles lose all tension, the ligaments have to take the strain. Invest in a decent bed and it will pay dividends in improved sleep. If you share a bed with your partner, check that it is big enough and able to accommodate your different body weights. Where body weights vary dramatically it can be worthwhile buying two differently sprung mattresses that can be zipped together. In any event, there should be no central sag between two sleeping partners.

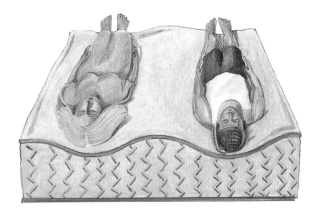

▲ *Where a couple share a double bed there should be no sag in the mattress between them.*

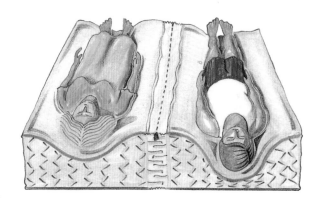

▲ *If a couple are of very different body weights, or if one prefers a firm mattress and the other a softer one, two differently sprung single mattresses can be zipped together to give each of them the support they need or prefer.*

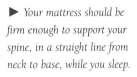

► *Your mattress should be firm enough to support your spine, in a straight line from neck to base, while you sleep.*

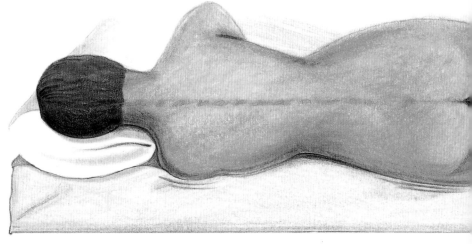

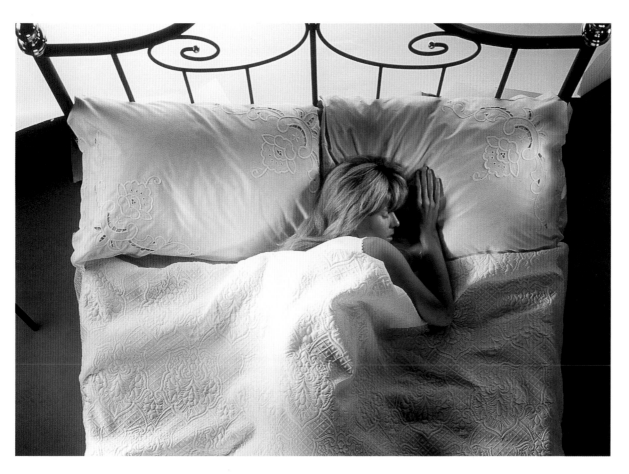

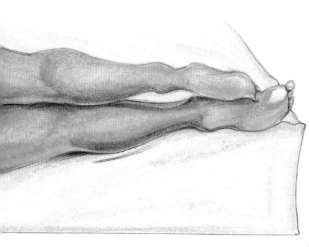

▲ *Whatever style of bed you choose, make sure your mattress provides the support and comfort you need.*

Lights Out

Research has shown that dimming the bedroom lights prior to sleep helps the body to begin its slowing-down process. So use a soft bedside light while getting ready for bed, and for reading before sleep. Also make sure that your room is dark enough for sleep: line drapes with thick, black fabric to shut out streetlights or early morning sun. Alternatively, if the dawn light falls across your pillow, change the position of the bed itself.

Snuggle Down

Pillows should be soft, whether filled with feathers or synthetic material. If you have allergies, feather pillows can aggravate them and give you a blocked nose. The pillow should support rather than raise your head. Too many pillows could give you a crick in the neck, and most people find sleeping without a pillow uncomfortable.

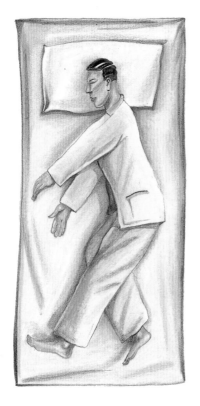

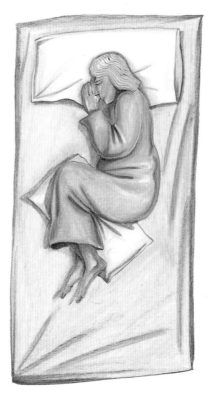

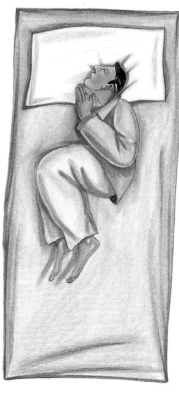

▲ *Check your posture in bed. If you are lying in an awkward position, you will be tense and find it difficult to sleep.*

▲ *Placing a pillow between the knees helps to avoid twisting the spine, and prevents aggravating any discomfort in the back.*

▲ *Sticking your neck out, even while sleeping, will cause strain.*

Curl up in Comfort

Getting into a comfortable position in bed is important, and the easier this is to do, the quicker you will fall asleep. If you experience any physical discomfort when lying in bed, your sleeping position may be responsible. Many people with back pain find that sleeping on their side with a small cushion or pillow between their knees reduces the twist on the spine. And think about tucking your chin in. We often unconsciously thrust our chins up and forward as we curl up, and this can create strain on the neck. Although you move around as you sleep, it helps to start out in comfort.

A Quiet Night

Although you can become accustomed to noise, and sleep through many sounds, perpetual half-waking at night can disturb your sleep and cause you to wake up still feeling tired. Too much silence, on the other hand, can make occasional noises seem very loud. Some people find that gentle background, or "white," noise works best. You can buy recordings of white noise, and research has shown that repetitive noises, such as a simulated heartbeat or waves breaking on the seashore, do help to induce sleep.

If noise is mainly caused by external factors, insulating the windows may help. Getting mad about noise only makes sleep less likely. Another remedy is earplugs. Those made of malleable wax block the ears very effectively, but sponge plugs that cut out less noise may be sufficient. If you know you are a "light sleeper," earplugs can make all the difference.

▶ *Earplugs can be a boon against nighttime disturbances, or when traveling and sleeping away from home.*

Even with earplugs, it is possible to hear the alarm, especially if it goes off at a regular hour, because your body will be expecting to rouse at this time.

Earplugs can be useful if you sleep alongside a noisy partner. They are also handy for occasional use, when the neighbors are having a party, for example, or when you are on vacation where nighttime noises are unfamiliar. The plugs must be comfortable to be effective, so try out various types. It could also take a while to get used to them.

Temperature and Fresh Air

The temperature in your bedroom should be around 65°F (18°C), and there should be an adequate supply of fresh air. This doesn't mean that you must open a window, if that increases draft and noise. Leaving the bedroom door open or ajar may be enough to allow air to circulate in the room.

Ionizers have improved the quality of sleep for many people, especially those with respiratory problems. An ionizer produces negative ions to counteract the positive ions present in a stuffy, polluted atmosphere. Air particles are electrically neutral but can acquire a positive charge from dust, electrical appliances, central heating, air conditioning, synthetic fibers, and pollution. Excessive positive ions are associated with headaches, irritability, and tension, whereas negative ions – created by running water, ocean waves, and lightning – make us feel alert and invigorated. If you think your bedroom is

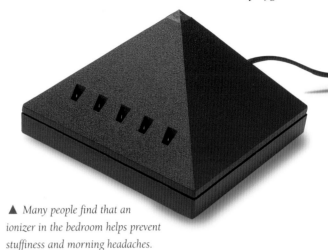

▲ *Many people find that an ionizer in the bedroom helps prevent stuffiness and morning headaches.*

stuffy and the air could be improved, putting a small ionizer in it may improve not just the quality of your sleep but also of your waking hours.

Although a warm room is conducive to sleep, being too hot will make you restless as your body attempts to cool down. The reverse is also true. If you go to bed chilly, or with cold feet, it takes you longer to relax and fall asleep. One of the reasons why a warm bath before bed is beneficial is because it gently heats the body prior to rest. Equally, if you are feeling hot and bothered, a bath can be a relaxing and soothing way to cool down.

Sharing a bed can cause temperature problems: one person may like to burrow beneath a voluminous comforter or layers of blankets, while the other is instantly too hot. One compromise is to have a bed large enough not to sleep virtually on top of one another, and each to have a quilt of different weight. Alternatively, compensate by wearing more, or less, nightclothes to reconcile individual temperature needs.

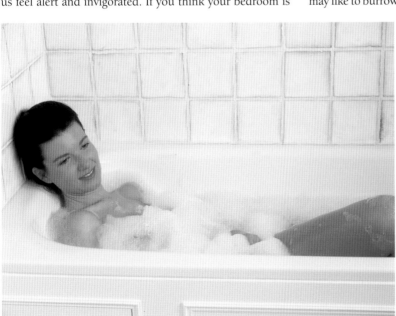

◀ *A warm bath helps relax muscles and can be conducive to sleep.*

The Role of Exercise

There is no doubt that people who exercise regularly sleep better. This doesn't mean excessive exercise, but a daily amount that helps release muscle tension and promote relaxation. Research has shown specific beneficial changes in sleep patterns between those who exercise and those who do not. Occasional, strenuous exercise, is not especially helpful, but regular exercise is. Experiments done with athletes showed that, after days when they took exercise, not only did they fall asleep more easily, they experienced longer periods of slow-wave sleep, which is the deeper and more restorative sleep.

Not Too Little, Not Too Much

The majority of people in middle age take too little exercise to meet their health needs. This coincides with a period of life when workloads and family demands are likely to be heavy, and there is little individual time for adequate physical exercise or relaxation. Generalized worries about work, finances, children, and relationships can mean that sleep is sacrificed and also becomes less easy to attain. A vicious circle can arise. So for the benefit of physical and mental health, of which sleep is part, some form of daily exercise is essential, whether this is simply walking home after work or a regular swim.

However, it is also known that strenuous exercise too close to the end of the day can be counterproductive in terms of sleep. This is especially so in the case of irregular, unaccustomed exercise. The busy executive's occasional game of squash after work is an obvious example, particularly if it is followed by several drinks at the bar afterwards. The heart rate increases and stays beating fast, and body temperature remains elevated after strenuous exercise of this type. The physical effect is too stimulating, and the body continues in an overheated and excited state for an extended period, making subsequent relaxation and sleep difficult.

Gentle Exercises

A useful part of your pre-bed routine is a series of gentle stretching and relaxation exercises. These relieve physical tension, realign muscles and ligaments, and reduce the possibility of stiffness and pain in bed. Yoga-based exercises are particularly good, and help create a relaxed approach to bedtime. Yoga breathing exercises can also assist the winding-down process at the end of the day, and a period of reflection or meditation is calming. Massage, or self-massage, of areas that are especially prone to tension – the shoulders, neck, and scalp, for example – is also beneficial before sleep.

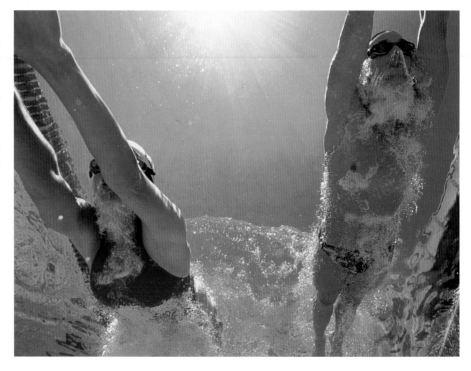

▶ *Choose a regular activity you enjoy – swimming is a good choice for many people – but avoid overstrenuous exercise late in the evening.*

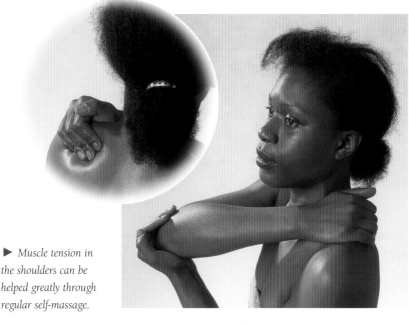

► *Muscle tension in the shoulders can be helped greatly through regular self-massage.*

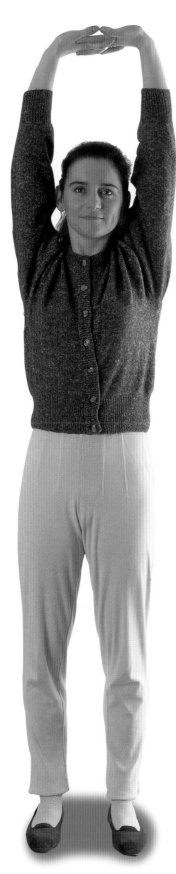

◄ *Even a simple stretch will relieve muscle tension if done on a regular basis.*

Regular Exercise

Exercise is extremely important for both a healthy waking life and healthy sleep. You need to find a form of exercise that you enjoy and that suits your lifestyle, so that you can fit it into your daily routine easily. Good forms of exercise include:

• **Swimming**
• **Aerobics**
• **Walking**
• **Cycling**

The health benefits of regular exercise are manifold. Exercise triggers the release of endorphins, the body's "pleasure hormones," and imparts a sense of well-being. It promotes oxygenation of the body's tissues, and keeps joints and muscles in good working order. If you find it difficult to maintain the willpower to exercise regularly, persuade a friend to join you, so that you can encourage each other and enjoy the exercise as a social activity. You will find that the physical sense of well-being, and the emotional benefits of knowing you have achieved your goal, will go a long way toward promoting good sleep.

Food and Drink

Where diet is concerned, sleep hygiene mostly concentrates on foods and drinks to avoid, especially in the period before sleep. Eating a large, rich meal and expecting to sleep well only hours afterwards is over-optimistic. Although many people like to eat their biggest meal in the evening, and make it a social occasion, it can contribute to over-stimulation of the gut and the body's response to the sheer quantity of the food can seriously challenge the ability to sleep. It is better to eat a light meal at the end of the day, with perhaps a pre-bed snack to avoid night hunger.

Daytime Drinks and Nightcaps

Drinking lots of coffee during the day is also unlikely to help you sleep well. If sleep is a problem, limit caffeine intake to two drinks a day, preferably before lunch. Switch to caffeine-free varieties, avoid colas and other carbonated drinks that contain caffeine, and choose fresh fruit juices and herbal

▲ *Freshly squeezed fruit juices are an alternative to tea, coffee, and other caffeine-based drinks such as colas.*

teas instead. Having a milky drink before bed is good, but avoid chocolate, as there is caffeine in that also. Although an alcoholic nightcap can seem effective in helping you to unwind, habitual use of alcohol in this way is not beneficial. The soporific effect of alcohol is most

▼ *A light meal is your best option at the end of the day.*

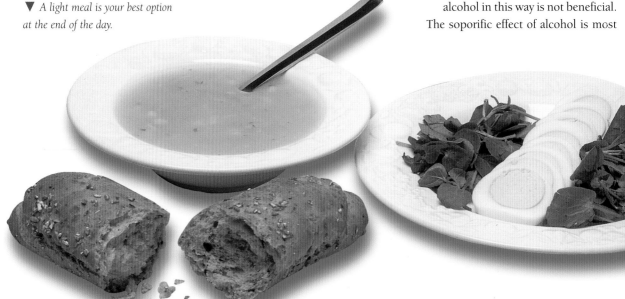

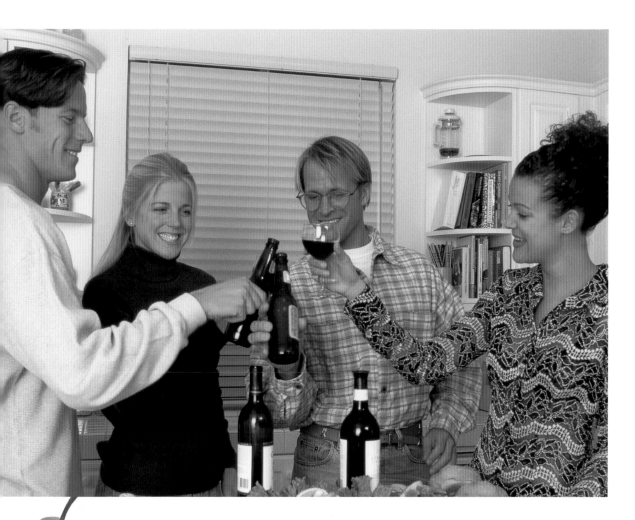

▲ Socializing with friends, and enjoying a drink, may be an important part of the way you relax, but don't overdo either late hours or the alcohol if you want to sleep well tonight.

pronounced when the drinker is already sleepy; it does nothing to help continued sleep. This is because alcohol disrupts normal sleep patterns. After its initial sedative effect, there is a rebound, and arousal is heightened, with an increase in REM (dreaming) sleep (see pages 34–35), and disturbance of the sleep cycle.

A "Good Night Out"

If alcohol and caffeine are combined, the sedative effects of the alcohol may be stronger than the alerting effects of the caffeine, and sleep may come easily. After a few hours, however, the sedative effects wear off, and the rebound effect of the alcohol combined with the alerting effects of the caffeine can find you wide-awake at 4 a.m. If cigarette smoking is added to this scenario, nicotine can contribute its stimulating effect to sleep problems. All of these factors may help to explain why we tend to sleep less well after a "good night out" than on other occasions!

All in all, therefore, if you have a pattern of sleep disturbances, or a long-term problem with sleep, you should review your daily intake of the stimulants, such as excessive caffeine from coffee or cola drinks, that can contribute to over-arousal and wakefulness.

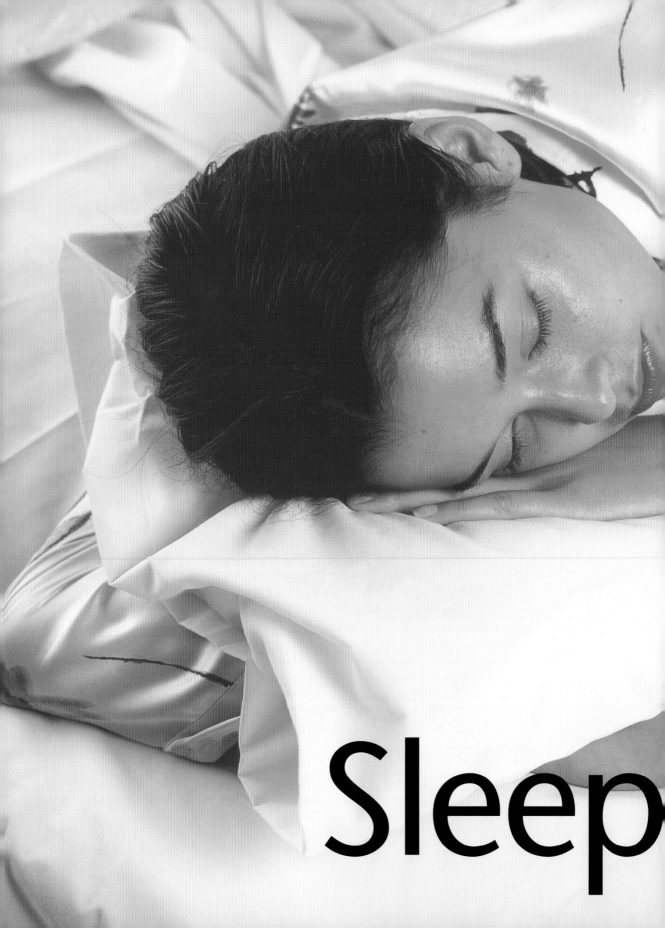

Sleep

Understanding how a sleep problem arises means knowing how sleep functions in the first place. It then becomes possible to figure out which simple, practical measures can help to solve the problem, and why certain remedies work for some people and not for others. Sleep is an individual process, and you need to know how it operates for you. As you come to recognize the factors that are causing the disruptions, you will be able to adjust and accommodate your body's demands for sleep.

Education

Functions of Sleep

One of the primary functions of sleep appears to be restorative, allowing time for physical and mental recuperation after the demands of the day. The cells of the body are continually being worn out and renewed, both day and night, but the process of cell renewal is greater during sleep.

Growth hormone, for example, is released mainly at night, and chiefly in conjunction with Stage 4 sleep (see pages 34–35). In children who receive extra growth hormone, because they don't produce enough to grow properly, the hormone works better when given at night.

Hormones for Wakefulness

Hormones are chemical messengers produced in one area of the body to have an effect elsewhere. They have a considerable role to play in our patterns of sleep and wakefulness. The pituitary gland secretes a hormone that stimulates the adrenal gland, situated near the kidneys, to produce corticosteroids, which enable us to feel awake. Corticosteroids reach peak levels in the morning, around the time we wake up.

The adrenal gland also produces another hormone for wakefulness: adrenalin. It is released in response to any extra demands placed upon us, and especially when we are frightened or under stress. It provides improved muscular power, in case we need it, and it uses up enormous energy reserves.

The Bodybuilders

These main hormones for wakefulness, corticosteroids and adrenalin, inhibit the body's ability to release other hormones that are necessary for cell growth and renewal. During sleep, production of the waking hormones diminishes, allowing the bodybuilding hormones to be released, and new growth to occur.

When the need for cell growth is increased – for example, during adolescence or pregnancy, or after exercise – both the duration of Stage 3 and Stage 4 sleep (see pages 34–35), and the overall amount of sleep are increased. This function of sleep is clearly in response to changing body demands.

Renewal of body cells also depends on making good use of the protein sources available. This process appears to be linked to the body's reduced metabolic rate when asleep, and its corresponding need for less oxygen. During this period of decreased oxygen consumption, the effects of the bodybuilding hormones are amplified. So sleep is obviously crucial to physical renewal.

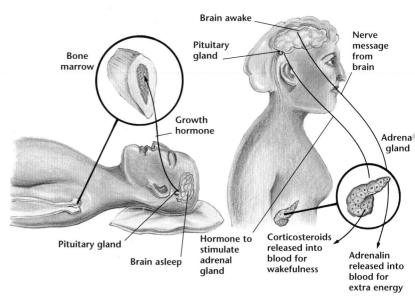

Brain awake · Pituitary gland · Nerve message from brain · Bone marrow · Growth hormone · Adrenal gland · Pituitary gland · Brain asleep · Hormone to stimulate adrenal gland · Corticosteroids released into blood for wakefulness · Adrenalin released into blood for extra energy

▲ *During sleep there is an increased production of growth hormone, which makes adequate sleep particularly important for growing children, especially adolescents.*

▲ *During the day, we produce larger quantities of corticosteroids and adrenalin, which prepare us for our waking activities.*

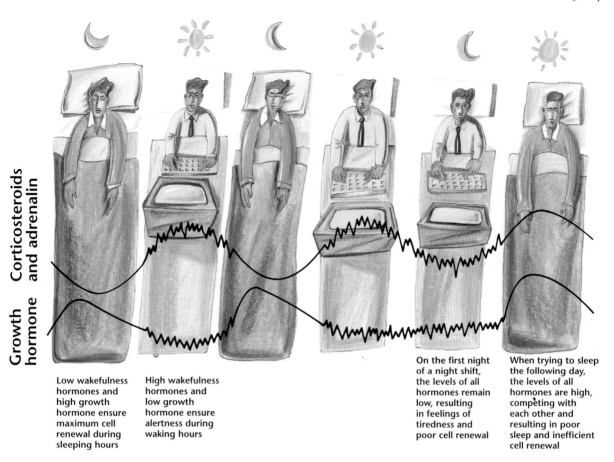

Corticosteroids and adrenalin

Growth hormone

Low wakefulness hormones and high growth hormone ensure maximum cell renewal during sleeping hours

High wakefulness hormones and low growth hormone ensure alertness during waking hours

On the first night of a night shift, the levels of all hormones remain low, resulting in feelings of tiredness and poor cell renewal

When trying to sleep the following day, the levels of all hormones are high, competing with each other and resulting in poor sleep and inefficient cell renewal

"Perchance to Dream"

But sleep doesn't just restore the body physically. Sleep, and in particular REM (dreaming) sleep (see pages 34–35), is considered to have a beneficial effect on various psychological functions. Dreaming is thought to be a way in which we process emotional experiences and other daytime material. The old saying about "sleeping on it" when faced with a difficult problem or decision is linked to this idea. This processing could also be a way of transferring recent memories into longer-term storage.

Everyone dreams, whether they think they do or not, because REM, or dreaming, sleep forms part of the sleep cycle. We may not remember our dreams when we wake up, or we may only recall them occasionally, but dreams have a purpose, and it exists for us all.

In his book *The Interpretation of Dreams*, published in 1901, and his work, Sigmund Freud, the father of modern psychoanalysis, set great store by what was apparently revealed in dreams. Subsequent analysts, including Carl

▲ *Hormones rise and fall in response to our contrasting day and night activities, and changing your sleeping pattern, such as at the start of a night shift, will inevitably cause problems as your body's hormone cycle adjusts.*

Jung, were equally convinced of the relevance of dreams to everyday life. Among other functions dreaming was thought to provide a safe outlet for the satisfaction of ordinarily suppressed urges. We could at least dream about all sorts of things that were impossible or unthinkable in real life.

Research done in the United States by Drs Fisher and Dement in the late 1950s, showed that depriving a group of volunteers of their dreams for five nights caused them to show a number of symptoms, including tension, anxiety, difficulty in concentration, irritability, and a tendency to hallucinate. When uninterrupted sleep patterns were resumed, there was an increase in the amount of REM sleep that occurred. There was no indication of long-term damage following the experiment.

Sleep Patterns

Sleep is not a single state, and most people are aware that there are different patterns, or phases, of sleep. During these phases, your body undergoes many functional changes, and the quality of your sleep varies.

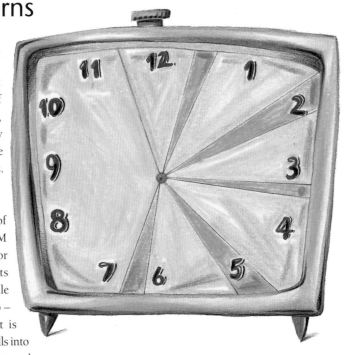

◀ *Throughout the night, our sleep is interspersed with periods of dreaming, or REM, sleep.*

Key

▨ Awake

▨ Non-REM sleep

▨ REM sleep

Non-REM Sleep

The two distinct phases of sleep are called non-REM and REM sleep, named for the rapid eye movements that occur at intervals while we sleep. Non-REM sleep – or orthodox sleep, as it is sometimes called – then falls into four different stages, interspersed by periods of REM sleep. Knowledge of these stages of sleep became possible when volunteers slept with electrodes attached to their heads to record their brain-wave patterns. Brain waves can be measured by an instrument called an electroencephalograph (EEG), which makes a recording of the electrical impulses given off by brain cells. The EEG printout shows distinct patterns indicative of the different stages of sleep.

Stage 1 non-REM sleep is the drowsy stage, where sleep is almost inevitable but not quite. During this stage of sleep you are vaguely aware of what is happening around you, and would equally be capable of nodding off completely, or of waking up instantly.

Stages 1 to 2

As you move from Stage 1 to Stage 2, you may experience a sudden jerk of the entire body which wakes you up. This is known as a "hypnagogic startle" – hypnagogic being the term that describes the process of falling asleep. These jerks are normal, although they may only happen infrequently. There is no reason to be concerned, as a hypnagogic startle appears to serve no purpose and is not indicative of any disorder. You can still be woken easily from Stage 2 sleep.

Stages 2 to 4

Sleep progresses from Stage 2 through the deeper level of Stage 3 to the deepest level, Stage 4. An EEG trace in Stage 4 shows deeper and longer brain waves, in contrast to the small, fast brain waves of lighter sleep. During Stage 4 sleep – sometimes referred to as deep-wave sleep – the breathing and heart rate become very stable. It would be difficult to wake during this stage of sleep without a powerful stimulus. But even in deepest sleep, your mind is able to process some information, and would respond to an urgent call to awaken, such as a baby's cry or a smoke alarm.

REM Sleep

Interspersed with non-REM sleep are periods of REM sleep, during which we dream. REM sleep is also known as paradoxical sleep, and it accounts for around 20 percent of all sleep. The recorded brain waves of REM sleep show a pattern that is closest to Stage 1 sleep. However, REM sleep is entirely different physically from all of the non-REM stages.

REM is an active state, even though you are asleep. Breathing and heart rate increase, and become much more irregular. The body uses more oxygen, indicating that more energy is being deployed, while kidney function, body reflexes, and patterns of hormone release all change. In contrast, the body's muscles are in a state of such deep relaxation that they are virtually paralyzed. The nerve impulses that normally travel freely up and down the spinal cord are effectively blocked. So although there is a lot of internal activity in terms of brain function and metabolism, there is limited movement during this phase. And many people have experienced the odd sensation of waking from a dream and being momentarily unable to move.

The most obvious symptom of REM sleep, however – from which it gets its name – is rapid eye movement, clearly visible under the closed eyelid. REM sleep occurs intermittently throughout the night, and the amount you need is controlled by the self-regulating mechanism of sleep. You cannot deliberately change your individual pattern of REM and non-REM sleep, except through the use of a number of drugs, which can affect both sleep patterns and the quality and depth of different stages of sleep. These include not only sleeping pills, but alcohol and other recreational drugs, such as cannabis.

Sleep Cycles

A sleep cycle is the time it takes to progress normally through all of the sleep stages, independent of the length of an individual stage, and including both REM and non-REM sleep. A baby born at full-term will have a sleep cycle of around 50 minutes, increasing to the adult length of 90 minutes by adolescence. This cycling of the different sleep stages explains why we sometimes wake up ready to go, and other times it is a struggle to get out of bed at the sound of the alarm.

▶ *In a sleep laboratory, each stage of sleep is recognizable by its quite distinct brain-wave patterns on an EEG trace. These occur and recur in sequence throughout our sleep cycle if it is uninterrupted, from Stage 1 through REM sleep.*

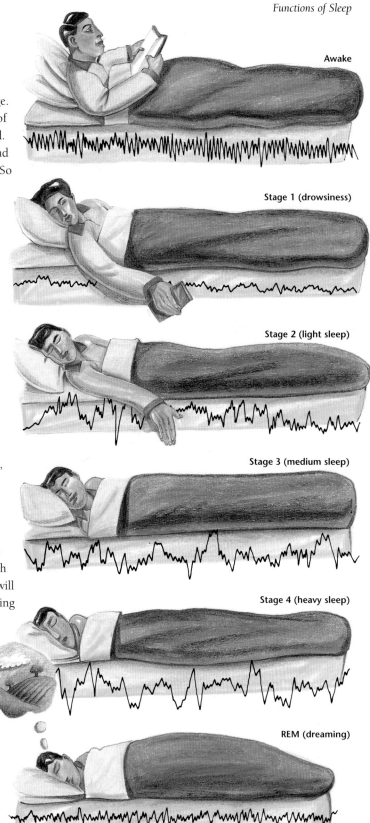

Awake

Stage 1 (drowsiness)

Stage 2 (light sleep)

Stage 3 (medium sleep)

Stage 4 (heavy sleep)

REM (dreaming)

Circadian Rhythms

Everyone has an internal "body clock" that functions on a roughly 24-hour cycle. This clock is also known as a biorhythm or a circadian rhythm, and it defines the cycles of your bodily functions: when you feel sleepy or wakeful, active or tired, when you want to eat, and less obviously, fluctuations in body temperature and hormone secretion. For example, your body temperature is dropping toward its daily minimum when you fall asleep, and is beginning to peak as you wake up. Levels of corticosteroids (see pages 32–33) diminish as you move toward bedtime, and build to a high level just before you wake.

The Body Clock

The body clock is thought to be regulated by the secretion of the hormone melatonin from the pineal gland (named for its pine-cone shape), which is situated in the upper part of the midbrain. This hormone is derived from serotonin, a naturally produced body chemical which plays a role in the transmission of nerve impulses, and has a function in controlling both mood and states of consciousness. Melatonin acts on the brain, helping to synchronize the day and night aspect of the circadian rhythm. Because humans have a diurnal rhythm – meaning that we are active during the hours of light – in contrast to nocturnal animals, the role of melatonin in that rhythm is regarded as important in the treatment of sleep disorders.

Our entire natural circadian rhythm is, in fact, closer to a 25-hour cycle than a 24-hour one. We maintain it on a 24-hour cycle through a process of constant readjustment, and it is the "clues" provided by regular mealtimes, bedtimes,

Relaxing before bedtime is very important in order to sleep well. Our body temperature steadily falls as we wind down from the day's activities in readiness for sleep.

The last meal of the day should be eaten at least two hours before going to bed. This avoids disrupting the body's rhythm.

Returning home at the end of the day, we begin to wind down, and our body temperature starts to lower.

Lunch is another important clue. Our body temperature continues to rise and usually reaches its peak by mid-afternoon, the time when most of us are fully alert.

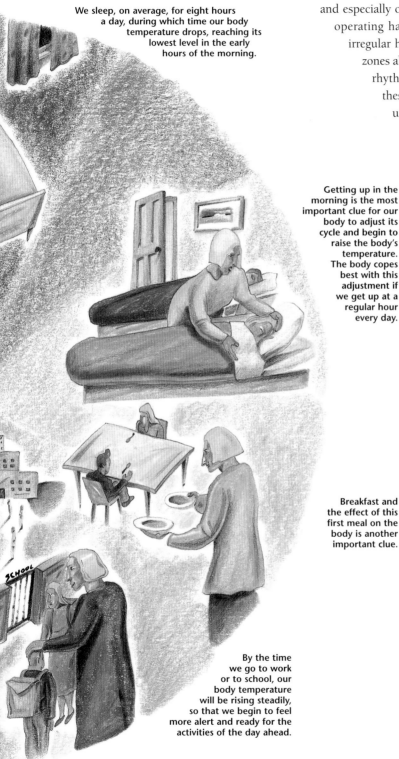

We sleep, on average, for eight hours a day, during which time our body temperature drops, reaching its lowest level in the early hours of the morning.

Getting up in the morning is the most important clue for our body to adjust its cycle and begin to raise the body's temperature. The body copes best with this adjustment if we get up at a regular hour every day.

Breakfast and the effect of this first meal on the body is another important clue.

By the time we go to work or to school, our body temperature will be rising steadily, so that we begin to feel more alert and ready for the activities of the day ahead.

and especially our getting-up time that keep our bodies operating happily on a 24-hour cycle. Continually irregular hours, shift work, and travel across time zones all upset our circadian rhythms. Disrupted rhythms mean disturbed sleep patterns, and these result in poor sleep at night and feeling under par during the day.

Highs and Lows

Probably the most obvious indicator of circadian rhythms is body temperature. It rises and falls throughout the day, and if you measured your temperature every hour, you would see the changes clearly. Temperature begins to rise before waking and continues to do so as the day progresses, reaching a peak in the afternoon, before it starts to decline. It reaches its lowest ebb in the early hours of the morning, which is the time of day when most deaths occur. Physical skill and intellectual performance rise and fall in line with body temperature changes. The higher our body temperature, the more alert we feel, and the more able we can be.

◄ *Our individual body clock, or circadian rhythm, is partly determined by the regularity of our waking and sleeping hours, with "clues" to the time of day being given by events like waking times and meal times.*

Sleep Disorders

The factors that influence sleep and wakefulness suggest how some sleep disorders can arise, and the steps you can take to remedy them.

If you keep irregular hours, sleeping and waking at different times every day, your circadian rhythms can only get confused. Bearing in mind the influence this has on body temperature, hormone secretions, and other functions, it is clear that entering a situation where the body is perpetually at odds with itself can be counterproductive to achieving a good night's sleep. It is very hard to get to sleep if your body temperature is high and you have numerous activating hormones, such as cortisol, whizzing around inside you. And this is only happening because your body thinks it is the middle of the afternoon, and not 11 o'clock at night, perhaps because you slept late this morning, having worked late last night and eaten a heavy meal at 9 p.m.

▼ *Numerous aspects of our busy lives can adversely affect our ability to sleep well. These can range from irregular sleeping hours, stress at work, depression, and worries over a health problem, to eating late at night or the over-stimulation of a late-night party.*

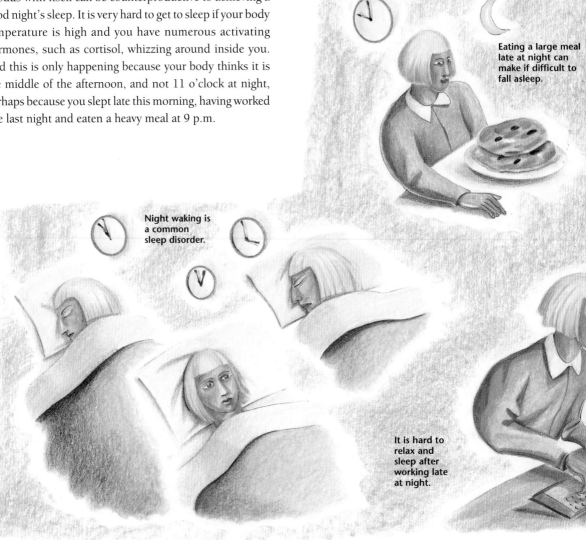

Eating a large meal late at night can make if difficult to fall asleep.

Night waking is a common sleep disorder.

It is hard to relax and sleep after working late at night.

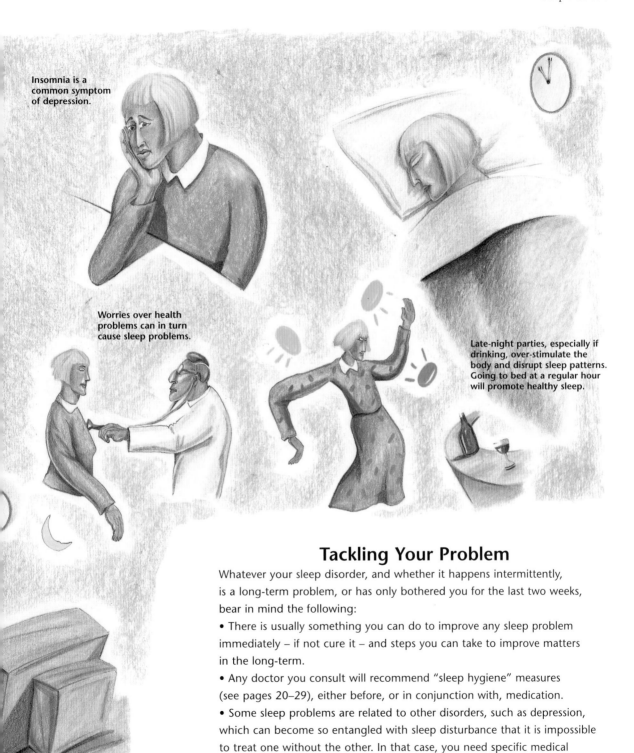

Insomnia is a
common symptom
of depression.

Worries over health
problems can in turn
cause sleep problems.

Late-night parties, especially if
drinking, over-stimulate the
body and disrupt sleep patterns.
Going to bed at a regular hour
will promote healthy sleep.

Tackling Your Problem

Whatever your sleep disorder, and whether it happens intermittently,
is a long-term problem, or has only bothered you for the last two weeks,
bear in mind the following:

• There is usually something you can do to improve any sleep problem
immediately – if not cure it – and steps you can take to improve matters
in the long-term.

• Any doctor you consult will recommend "sleep hygiene" measures
(see pages 20–29), either before, or in conjunction with, medication.

• Some sleep problems are related to other disorders, such as depression,
which can become so entangled with sleep disturbance that it is impossible
to treat one without the other. In that case, you need specific medical
treatment relevant to your individual circumstances.

• However trivial you might think your poor sleep is, it can seriously impair
your enjoyment of life and is worth seeking to improve.

Insomnia

Insomnia is the inability to sleep, whether this is an inability to fall asleep, waking up during the night and being unable to return to sleep, or waking too early in the morning. It is a sleep disorder that is estimated to affect around 1 in 3 adults at some time during their lives. There are three categories of insomnia: transient, short-term, and chronic.

How Bad is Your Insomnia?

Transient insomnia can occur in response to an event – such as moving house or problems at work – or in anticipation of some circumstance. It only lasts a couple of nights and resolves itself with little or no trouble. Short-term insomnia lasts on and off for up to three weeks. It too generally happens in response to an external factor, which is probably of greater severity than the cause of transient insomnia. A death in the family, job change, serious illness, and relationship breakdown are the type of events that can lead to short-term insomnia. Chronic insomnia occurs where sleep is disturbed for more than three weeks. Around 15 percent of the population estimate their sleep disorders to be chronic.

Causes of Sleeplessness

Insomnia is the symptom of a problem, which is to some degree reassuring, because in diagnosing the underlying difficulty, a solution can be found. The main causes are linked to our lifestyle: erratic hours, use of stimulants, such as caffeine and nicotine, consumption of alcohol, and lack of exercise, for example. External factors, such as traffic noise, which you may hardly notice but which wakes you intermittently all night, can contribute to poor sleep. Persistent stress is also a factor, and when psychological problems move into depression, insomnia is a classic symptom, especially when there is early-morning waking.

Of course, there are people who never have sleep problems. And you may only be susceptible at particular life stages or under certain conditions, but the one thought to hang on to if you are experiencing difficulties with sleep is that most causes of insomnia are learned habits, and can therefore be unlearned, although this can take a little time.

For example, many people anticipate being unable to sleep if under stress, and need to learn ways of diffusing this anxiety so that it does not affect their sleep. Others need to

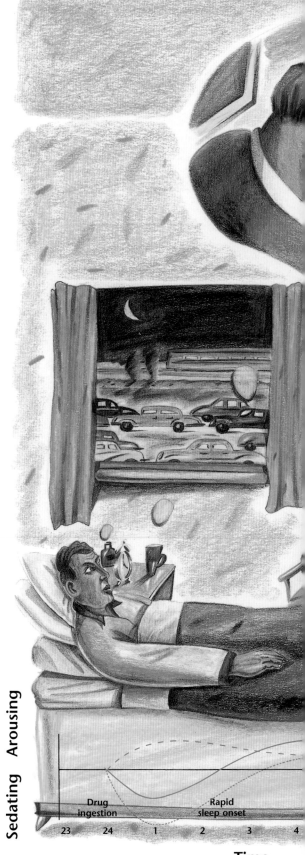

Arousing

Sedating

Drug ingestion

Rapid sleep onset

23 24 1 2 3 4

Time

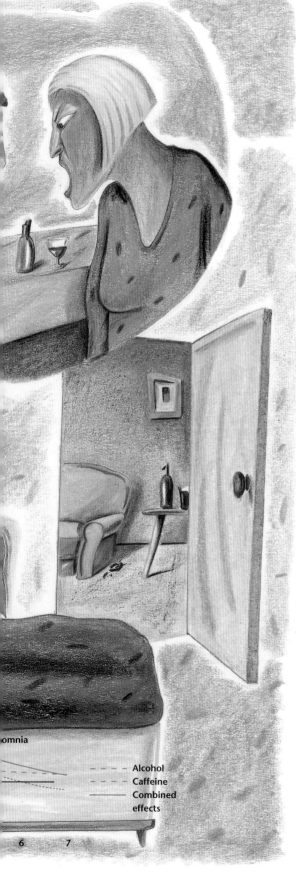

omnia

——— ——— — Alcohol
– – – Caffeine
——— Combined
effects

6   7

adopt relaxation techniques to avoid panicking or getting angry when sleep doesn't happen immediately – responses that decrease the chance of falling asleep easily. Worrying about not sleeping, and being unable to perform well at work, is a frequent problem. This concern transfers itself to the bedroom, which instead of being a cue to sleep, becomes a cue to anxiety. If this is your problem, you may find that you sleep perfectly well in places and at times where sleep is not expected.

It is also important to eliminate external factors that may be contributing to a sleep problem. Noise and light have already been mentioned, but physical discomfort or pain can profoundly affect the quality of sleep. A person changes position during sleep about 40 times on average. Generally, the less you move, the more restful sleep is. When you experience discomfort or pain, however, you may move more, or the movement that you make may increase the distress, and wake or part-wake you continuously through the night. The quality of your bed can play a much bigger role in this than you might think. During acute episodes of pain, take a painkiller, but check that it contains no stimulant: caffeine is often added to aspirin, paracetamol, and codeine. If you suffer from chronic (long-term) pain, consult your doctor to obtain the appropriate treatment.

Involuntary Movements

Brief muscle contractions that cause the legs to jerk at 30-second intervals for an hour or so, on and off during the course of the night, can severely disrupt sleep. This "periodic limb movement" generally affects older people, and is often associated with a daytime problem of restless legs. Iron-deficient anemia can sometimes be the cause, and adjustment to diet, with possibly an iron supplement, can help. Gentle evening exercise to stretch the muscles and ease tension, followed by a warm bath, is also beneficial.

◀ *Insomnia can become a problem for a number of reasons, such as worrying about arguments with work colleagues or loved ones. A poor sleeping environment, with a lot of nighttime noise, can also adversely affect sleep. The combination of late-night alcohol and coffee consumption is a common cause of transient insomnia, the alcohol often helping initial sleep but the combined effects resulting in night waking and the inability to return to restful sleep.*

Sleep Apnea and Snoring

Snoring is not only extremely irritating to a sleeping partner, but can be the symptom of a greater problem for the snorer: sleep apnea, meaning breathing stoppage. Sleep apnea is estimated to affect around 2 percent of the population and is a major cause of daytime sleepiness.

When we are awake we breathe primarily through our noses, and in this way the air inhaled passes gently over the soft palate into the lungs. When we breathe through our mouths, the passage of air is less controlled, and tends to pass through the back of the throat in a rush. If we breathe through our mouths when asleep, the vibrating of the soft tissues at the back of the throat produces the noise of snoring. This process is exacerbated by the fact that, during sleep, the muscles at the back of the throat are highly relaxed, so that the soft tissues are less supported than usual and can vibrate with varying degrees of loudness. The loudest snore on record peaked at 93 decibels, which is comparable with heavy city traffic!

Sleep apnea arises when the air passages narrow so much during sleep that breathing is blocked. Fortunately sleep doesn't obliterate the urge to breathe, and when the blockage occurs and the respiratory centers of the brain register that the oxygen supply has gone, the person wakes momentarily and regains control of the air passages. This process – of which the sufferer may be completely unaware – can be heard in the characteristic breathing pattern of someone with sleep apnea: loud snoring, interspersed with silence, followed by a particularly noisy inhalation and probably some body movement

It is easy to see that this constant waking or half-waking has a detrimental effect on normal sleep patterns. But it is more serious than that. Research recently published in Sweden demonstrated that people with sleep apnea have a threefold higher risk of coronary heart disease. That makes apnea a bigger risk factor in heart disease than high blood pressure or high blood cholesterol.

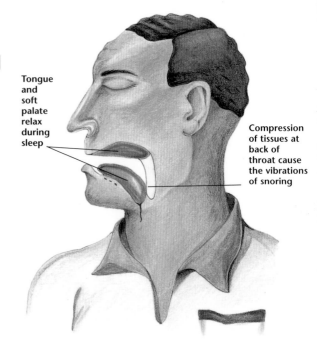

Tongue and soft palate relax during sleep

Compression of tissues at back of throat cause the vibrations of snoring

▲ *Snoring occurs when we breathe through our mouths during sleep and the soft tissues and muscles at the back of the throat are so relaxed that they block slightly and vibrate against each other.*

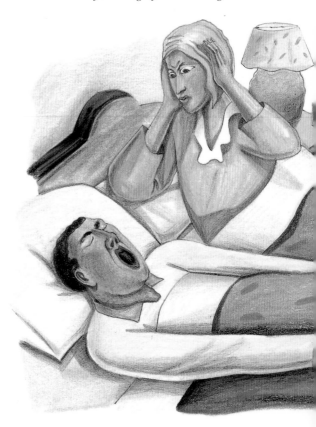

The Problem of Snoring: Who Snores and Why?

• Numerous factors contribute to snoring and sleep apnea. Gender is significant: around 41 percent of men are snorers, compared with 28 percent of women. There are possible links with the hormone testosterone in men and progesterone in women. Research has also shown that snoring gets progressively worse in men after the age of 20, while in women this does not occur until the age of 40.

• When excessive snoring, with or without apnea, occurs in children, it is usually due to enlarged tonsils and adenoids. The snoring may be the most obvious symptom, but these children can also be cranky, and find it difficult to settle down or learn, because of persistent over-tiredness – or be difficult to manage because they are hyperactive. There can be a history of night wakings, and possibly problems with bedwetting. If this seems a familiar picture, discuss the matter with your doctor.

• Obesity and being overweight increase the probability of snoring. Increased body fat is also situated around the airways, and combined with the muscle relaxation during sleep, contributes to the narrowing of the passages. If there is a lot of fat around the neck, this will exacerbate the problem. Weight loss will make a big, and immediate, difference.

• Smoking means breathing in substances that irritate the sensitive lining of the airways. This can cause excessive production of mucus and the resultant catarrh, forcing smokers to adopt the habit of breathing through their mouths, which continues at night and makes snoring much more likely. Smokers are twice as likely to snore as nonsmokers.

• During a cold, when the nose is blocked, snoring becomes more common, but this usually passes once the cold has gone.

• For people who suffer from hayfever or allergies, a blocked nose may be a continual problem, causing mouth breathing and snoring. Synthetic pillows, and allergy-free bedding can help, and the judicious use of antihistamines may be beneficial. Sleeping with an ionizer in the bedroom can be highly effective.

• Drinking alcohol heavily and regularly makes snoring much worse and contributes to the possibility of sleep apnea. The muscles of the airway, already relaxed by sleep, will be further affected. Even those who never snore will probably do so after a few drinks, while those who snore anyway will snore more.

• The position in which you sleep also affects your likelihood of snoring. Sleeping on the back makes snoring worse, because the jaw tends to fall open while compressing the back of the throat. If sleeping on your side means you continually roll over, try pushing a pillow into the lower part of your back. Alternatively, many people have found that elevating the head of the bed a little, by propping it up with a brick or telephone directory, is helpful.

Most of the reasons for snoring and sleep apnea can be simply addressed. However, if the problem is caused by injury or damage to the nasal passages – following a broken nose, for example – it may be necessary to have the damage repaired surgically, and you should consult an ear, nose, and throat specialist.

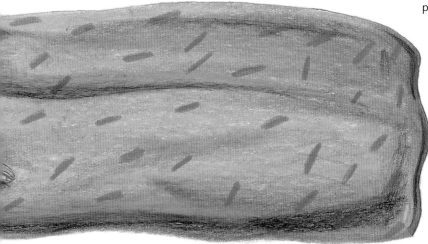

◄ *Snoring can also cause insomnia in the snorer's partner, by keeping him or her awake at night.*

Narcolepsy

Narcolepsy is a chronic and debilitating sleep disorder, which causes excessive daytime sleepiness (EDS), cataplexy (or sudden loss of muscle tone), sleep paralysis on falling asleep or on waking, and visual and auditory hallucinations on dozing or waking. Fortunately, only 11 percent of sufferers experience all four symptoms. It was recently discovered that people with narcolepsy have a sleep pattern that differs substantially from that of non-sufferers. The REM phase normally occurs after about 90 minutes of regular sleep. In people with narcolepsy, however, REM generally happens within 10 minutes of falling asleep. As a result of this rapid onset of the REM, sufferers can experience hallucinations.

EDS

By far the most common symptom of narcolepsy is EDS, and it is also the most difficult to treat. The sensation of sleepiness is irresistible, and people with narcolepsy have been known to fall asleep while walking, eating, and in mid-conversation. Attacks usually last around 30 minutes, after which a sufferer may awake feeling refreshed. But this sensation is generally shortlived, because within a couple of hours another attack occurs. Most sufferers feel drowsy when they wake in the mornings and a persistent feeling of fatigue can last all day. Up to 80 percent experience decreased alertness lasting a few seconds or a few minutes at a time, which is potentially dangerous, depending on their activity.

The Effects of Narcolepsy

A study carried out by the State University, Pennsylvania, discovered how badly sufferers' lives could be affected by narcolepsy. Fifty eight percent of participants recalled how they had fallen asleep during class and their school results had been adversely affected; 36 percent had been thought lazy or indifferent by their teachers. At work, 92 percent had experienced problems; 24 percent were forced to leave their jobs; and 18 percent were fired because of their illness. In relationships, 72 percent reported that narcolepsy had caused problems in their families, and 20 percent indicated that it had contributed to their divorce. Sexual problems were also common, including loss of libido and impotence. Unsurprisingly, many sufferers reported low self-esteem, chronic anxiety, and depression.

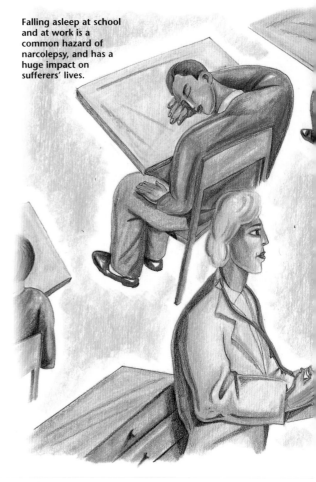

Falling asleep at school and at work is a common hazard of narcolepsy, and has a huge impact on sufferers' lives.

Diagnosis and Treatments

Recognition of the disease is not always easy, and inadequate or inaccurate diagnosis can retard treatment. When other conditions, such as low thyroid, multiple sclerosis, brain tumor, and even sleep apnea, which can be a cause of EDS, have been ruled out, sleep laboratory tests provide the most accurate diagnosis.

There is no cure for narcolepsy, and sufferers need to work out lifestyle changes, with the help of their doctor, in order to work around their condition. A structured sleep pattern is often recommended, with scheduled "nap" periods during the day, in an effort to increase general alertness and avoid unexpected naps. There is much that can be done, with sympathetic help, to manage the problem.

Other treatments have included the use of stimulants, such as caffeine or amphetamines, but these produced their own problems. Most sufferers found that although their

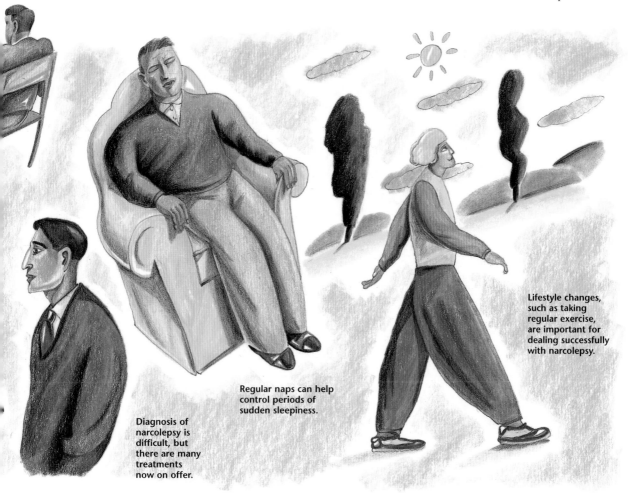

Diagnosis of narcolepsy is difficult, but there are many treatments now on offer.

Regular naps can help control periods of sudden sleepiness.

Lifestyle changes, such as taking regular exercise, are important for dealing successfully with narcolepsy.

sleepiness was controlled to a certain extent, they had to tolerate unwanted side-effects associated with the drugs, which also became less effective over time. There was also a strong risk of dependency, especially in the case of amphetamines. Where symptoms include cataplexy, however, antidepressants have sometimes proved useful.

The outlook for sufferers is, however, promising. Research continues and new treatments are becoming available. A recent drug, tested for four years in France, is non-amphetamine and non-addictive. It seems to increase wakefulness and restores a normal pattern of daytime alertness. It also appears to be effective in treating cataplexy, and does not disrupt nighttime sleep. The only significant side-effect to emerge after two large-scale studies was headache symptoms reported in a number of users.

Narcolepsy is a serious sleep disorder, and like many problems associated with the mysterious world of sleep, it

▲ *Unsurprisingly, narcolepsy has a major impact on the lives of its sufferers, from school age onward. There are, however, many things that can be done to control the condition. Consulting a doctor is essential, but self-help methods are also useful. Scheduling naps into the daily routine and taking regular exercise, for example, can both help to some extent.*

is not simply solved. Although the sufferer has no difficulty falling asleep – quite the reverse – the feelings of daytime fatigue and irritability are, ironically, similar to those of the insomniac, or of the sufferer from sleep apnea. In all cases, self-care is important, and lifestyle changes may be imperative, which is why a greater understanding of sleep and its functions can be beneficial.

Children

Adequate sleep is crucial in enabling children to grow and develop properly. Although their requirements change, children generally need much more sleep than adults. This is partly to give their bodies the opportunity to create and benefit from growth hormone, which is secreted at night. And at certain times children need additional sleep, because of a growth spurt, or recovery from illness, or because they are becoming more active.

The sleep habits learned now will last your children for the rest of their lives. It is worth remembering this when arguments arise about bedtimes. "It's for your own good" is self-evident – although probably better left unsaid! There is, as with all parenting, room for negotiation and compromise on occasions, but children must have adequate sleep to function, to feel good, and to be pleasant to be around. A tired child is not only likely to be cranky, but can also exhibit symptoms of hyperactivity, as the hormones for wakefulness, cortisol and adrenalin, go into overdrive to compensate for lack of sleep. Adhering to, or introducing, good sleep habits promotes balanced functioning, and can resolve a variety of child-health problems.

▶ *Some babies sleep well within weeks of birth, but the majority will need time to learn how, and their parents to teach them.*

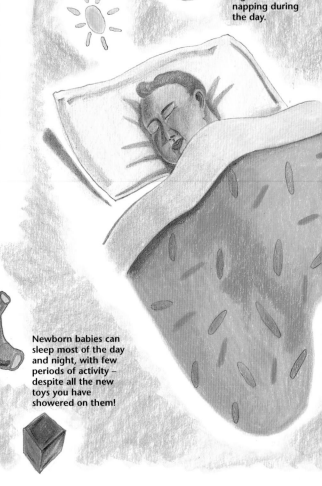

At 1–2 years old, a child will usually sleep peacefully throughout the night as well as napping during the day.

Newborn babies can sleep most of the day and night, with few periods of activity – despite all the new toys you have showered on them!

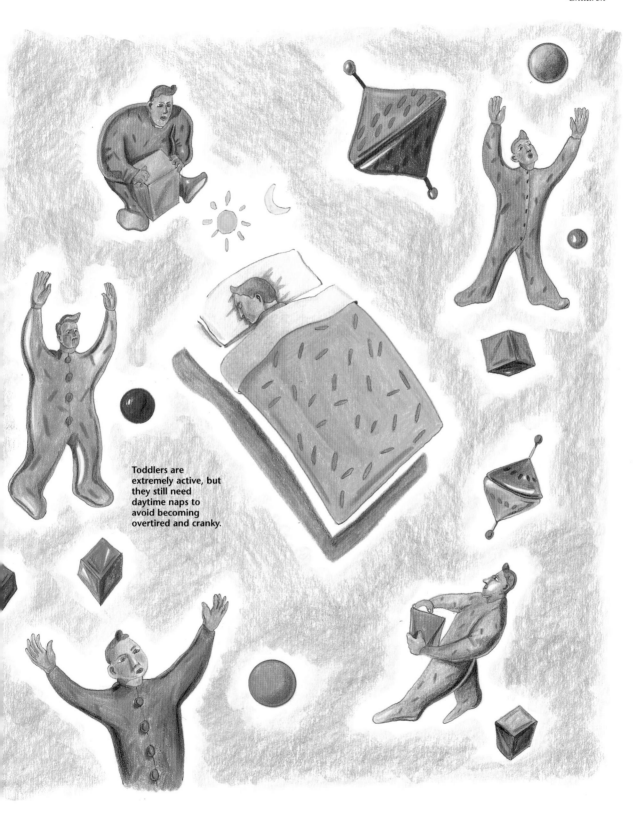

Toddlers are
extremely active, but
they still need
daytime naps to
avoid becoming
overtired and cranky.

A New Baby's Sleep Patterns

There is evidence that sleep patterns start in the womb. From about six or seven months of pregnancy, the unborn baby shows signs of REM sleep, and from around seven or eight months, non-REM sleep. In babies, these are also referred to as active sleep and quiet sleep, and by birth both states of sleep are well-established.

Active and Quiet Sleep

In the newborn, states of active and quiet sleep are both easy to see. During active sleep, you can observe the baby's eyes moving about under the eyelids; the baby makes little movements or twitches, breathes irregularly, and may smile briefly. In quiet sleep, infants lie very still, and breathe so quietly and deeply that they sometimes appear not to be breathing at all. A baby may occasionally jerk, or "startle," during quiet sleep, and sometimes makes sucking movements and noises with the mouth.

In contrast to older children, the newborn's non-REM sleep is not yet divided into four stages (see pages 34–35). Full-term babies spend about 50 percent of their sleep time in REM, or active, sleep, while premature babies spend around 80 percent of sleep time in REM. Non-REM sleep requires a certain amount of brain maturation, which occurs during the first few months of life. This explains why, during the early weeks of life, a baby's sleep pattern is so haphazard, and introducing any sort of routine takes time.

At birth, when a baby falls asleep, he or she enters REM sleep immediately. At around three months of age, this changes to a pattern of non-REM sleep first. That pattern is then set for life. In babies and young children, however, there is a rapid descent (around 10 minutes) from drowsiness to stage 4 sleep, which is why the young fall asleep so heavily, so fast. Stage 4 sleep then lasts for about an hour.

How Long Should a Baby Sleep?

The biggest difference between the sleep cycles of babies and adults is their length. An adult cycle is approximately 90 minutes; a baby's sleep cycle is only around 50 minutes. This means that roughly every hour there is a transitional state in a baby's sleep pattern, which may include a brief awakening, and a period of REM sleep with a degree of activity. As long as a baby is able to resettle, the return to a deeper stage of sleep will occur naturally and full wakening should not occur.

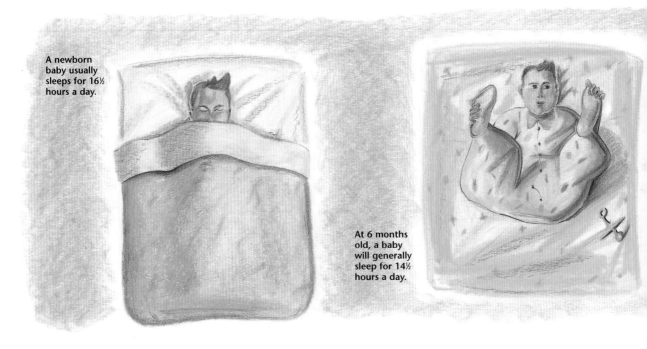

A newborn baby usually sleeps for 16½ hours a day.

At 6 months old, a baby will generally sleep for 14½ hours a day.

Newborn Babies

A typical sleep requirement for a newborn baby is around 16½ hours in a 24-hour period. In fact, immediately after birth a baby may sleep more or less all the time to recover from the physical demands of labor. By about four weeks of age, sleep drops to around 15½ hours out of 24; and at six months to around 14½ hours, with a larger proportion of sleep (1–11 hours) occurring at night. By the age of two, this changes again to around 13 hours – with approximately 12 hours sleep at night and around an hour's nap a day, or some similar pattern.

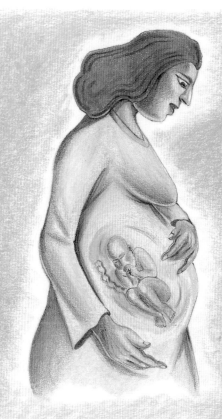

A baby's sleep patterns start to develop in the womb.

◀ *A baby's sleep patterns first develop in the womb, and both REM and non-REM sleep cycles are established by the time the baby is born. A newborn baby sleeps for around 16½ hours. By six months, the baby will be more active and only sleep for around 14½ hours. At a year old, he or she is much more alert and sleeps for 13¾ hours, which drops by another ½ hour by the age of 18 months.*

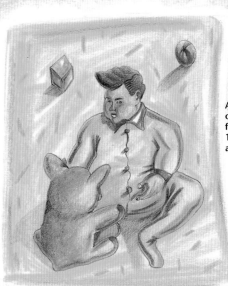

A 1-year-old sleeps for around 13¾ hours a day.

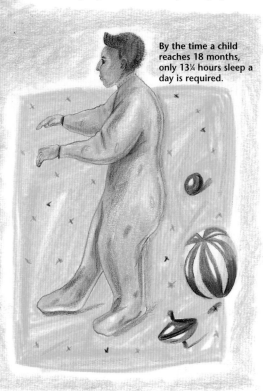

By the time a child reaches 18 months, only 13¼ hours sleep a day is required.

Developing Good Sleep Habits

Because a baby's neurological control of his or her sleep patterns lacks maturity, a regular day and night sleep routine is difficult to introduce at first. However, as soon as feeding is established and a baby has settled down after the birth, you can begin introducing clues that enable your baby to learn the difference between sleeping at night and during the day, and make it possible for him or her to sleep through the night after about three months of age.

First of all, give your baby the chance to learn how to go to sleep occasionally without your help. Avoid holding the baby – and feeding, rocking, or singing – until he or she falls asleep. Whether this is during the day or night – seductive though it is to nurture your baby to sleep – making it an unvarying routine means that the baby will come to rely on a certain set of circumstances that include your proximity in order to fall asleep. Don't be tempted to pick up and rearrange your baby every time he or she stirs. Some babies need to grumble a little while they settle and get comfortable, so leave them to it. But never allow your baby to cry for longer than 10 minutes, or to become thoroughly agitated, or the baby will conclude that going to bed is not a positive experience.

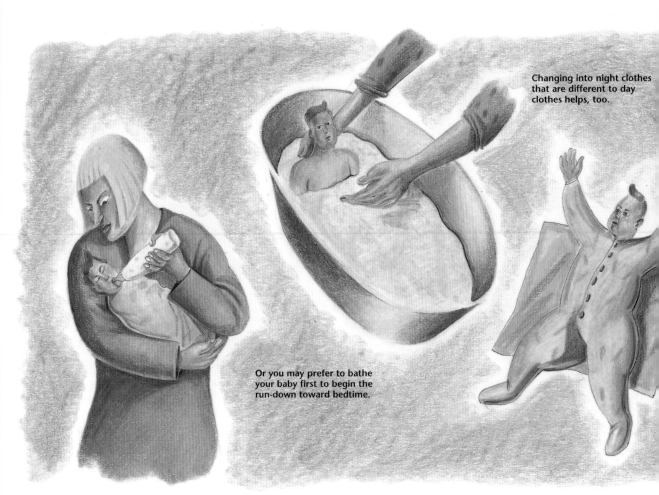

Changing into night clothes that are different to day clothes helps, too.

Or you may prefer to bathe your baby first to begin the run-down toward bedtime.

A final evening feed can be the trigger to the start of a bedtime routine.

Time for Bed

It is a good idea to introduce bedtime at a relatively young age. Like the sleep hygiene recommended for adults (see pages 20–29), babies need clues to teach them about day and night. From about six months, if your baby is happily eating solid food during the day, constant night feedings should be a thing of the past. Introduce a regular bedtime routine, perhaps consisting of supper, bathtime, pyjamas, a last drink, cuddle, and finally book time. Whatever routine you introduce, it must come to mean one inevitable thing: bed and sleep. After this, any nighttime communication should be very low-key and not involve leaving the bedroom until the following morning.

Even if this seems like an impossibility as you contemplate your newborn, the process of learning over the next six months will pay dividends in the long term, especially when you consider that you are giving your baby a skill for life: the ability to go to bed and sleep easily.

▼ *Like everyone else, babies need "clues" to establish their waking and sleeping patterns, especially when they are first learning to adjust to day and night. Creating a bedtime routine helps them to learn one set of clues which they can associate with sleeping.*

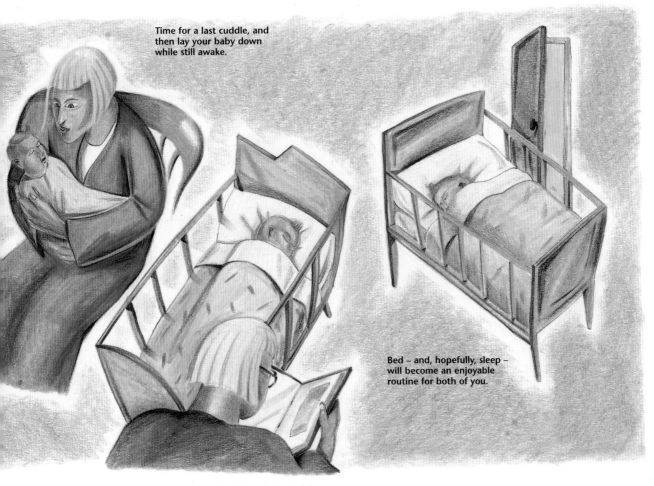

Time for a last cuddle, and then lay your baby down while still awake.

Bed – and, hopefully, sleep – will become an enjoyable routine for both of you.

Look at a picture book together; as the child grows older, read a nighttime story.

51

Dreams, Terrors, and Bedwetting

During REM, or dreaming, sleep, the body is in such a state of deep muscle relaxation that movement is impossible. If the dream is disturbing, a child may wake fully during the state of partial arousal that normally marks the transition from REM to non-REM sleep. The child might then call out or cry in fright at the memory of the dream. Whether or not your child can tell you about it will depend partly on his or her age, but a child of any age will be reassured by your presence and comfort following a bad dream, especially as the fear may persist for some time and delay a return to sleep. Nightmares, if they happen, tend to occur in the second half of the night, when dreams are strongest.

Night Terrors

Night terrors are different. They occur during a partial arousal from very deep, non-dreaming sleep. A child may scream and thrash about during a night terror, which is more likely to occur during the first four hours of sleep. There are signs of very obvious fright, anger, and perhaps confusion, which disappear if the child actually wakes. Offering comfort during a night terror is counterproductive and may aggravate the situation. Once the episode has passed, the child will rapidly return to sleep and have no memory of the event on waking.

Bedwetting

By about 2½ years of age, around 50 percent of children are dry at night; about 75 percent by age 3 years; and almost all by age 4. Staying dry at night depends on a number of factors: being dry during the day; being able to respond to bladder signals even when sleeping; maturation in the

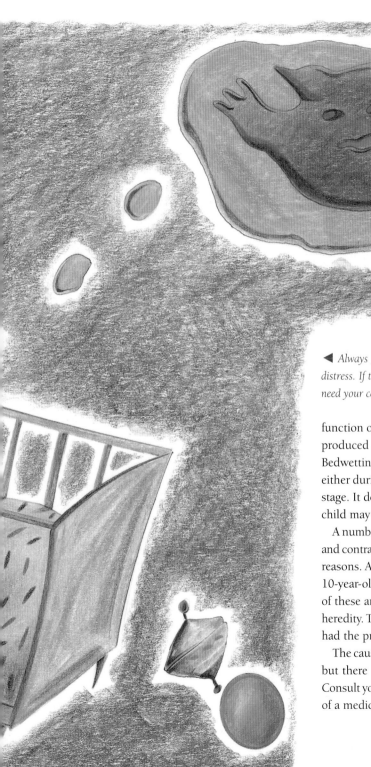

◄ *Always go to a child if they wake in distress. If they have had a nightmare, they will need your comfort and reassurance.*

function of the hormones that reduce the amount of urine produced at night; and the bladder's capacity to hold urine. Bedwetting tends to occur during the first third of the night, either during or just after an arousal from a non-REM sleep stage. It does not occur during dreaming sleep, although a child may dream about urinating because the bed is wet.

A number of children have difficulty becoming dry at night and contrary to popular opinion, this is seldom for emotional reasons. Around 15 percent of 5-year-olds and 5 percent of 10-year-olds still wet their beds regularly. About 60 percent of these are boys, and the single biggest factor is probably heredity. The incidence increases to 45 percent if one parent had the problem, and 75 percent if both did.

The causes of bedwetting (nocturnal enuresis) are various, but there are effective approaches to solving the problem. Consult your family doctor to rule out the unlikely possibility of a medical problem, and to obtain advice.

Body Changes and Changing Sleep Requirements

The quantity and quality of sleep we need changes as we progress through life. A toddler, a teenager, a pregnant or menopausal woman, and an octogenarian all have different sleep requirements. When we are sick or when we travel, our sleep demands alter. It is important to take these variations into account when tackling a sleep problem – bearing in mind that, whatever your age or physical condition, you can make positive adjustments to your sleep patterns.

Although it is possible to make recommendations about how much sleep each individual needs at a particular stage of their life, the best guide to how much you need is how you feel the following day. For example, if you are sleeping 10 hours a night and always feel lethargic when you wake, you may need less sleep and not more. Or you may find that you can sleep badly for a number of nights without really noticing it before needing several nights of going to bed on time, or slightly earlier, to catch up. And many people find that when on holiday, they sleep extensively and still feel as if they need more, as if they are compensating for some long-term sleep deficit. Sleep is such a subjective process and whether or not we need more or less sleep needs evaluating over a period of weeks rather than days.

▶ *From newborn to adolescent, from pregnancy to menopause, from time zone to time zone – our sleep needs change throughout our lives.*

After puberty the body undergoes an enormous acceleration in growth, and this affects the amount of sleep that adolescents require.

Newborn babies need lots of sleep to recover from the physical demands of labor.

54

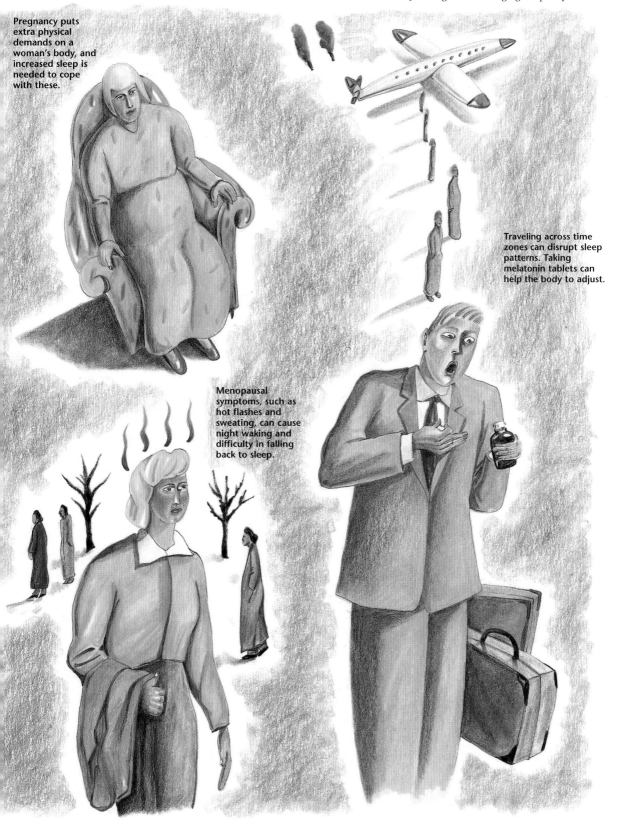

Pregnancy puts extra physical demands on a woman's body, and increased sleep is needed to cope with these.

Traveling across time zones can disrupt sleep patterns. Taking melatonin tablets can help the body to adjust.

Menopausal symptoms, such as hot flashes and sweating, can cause night waking and difficulty in falling back to sleep.

From Toddlers to Teenagers

A toddler (1–2 years) should normally sleep continuously through the night. Even if sleep patterns change occasionally, reversion to good sleep habits should happen with ease. A child of 18 months should be asleep for around 14 hours a day, with the longest sleep at night. A 12-hour night and a 2-hour nap during the day would be one good pattern.

Even if a toddler seems to be managing on much less sleep, it could be inadequate, and it would be advisable to increase the amount. It is tempting to think that a child who is kept awake all day will sleep better at night. This is not

the case: chronic over-tiredness causes the child's body to compensate with increased levels of "wakefulness" hormones (see pages 32–33), which make settling down and sleeping at night more difficult.

The Impact of School

When children start school, they face additional demands, both physically and emotionally. Many children need more sleep, or slightly earlier bedtimes, to help them cope with this transitional stage. It is therefore important to insist on reasonable sleeping time, with a regular routine and fixed bedtime hour, at least on school nights. Even so, during the

▼ *The amount of sleep children need gradually decreases as they grow older, and it is important to understand these changing requirements.*

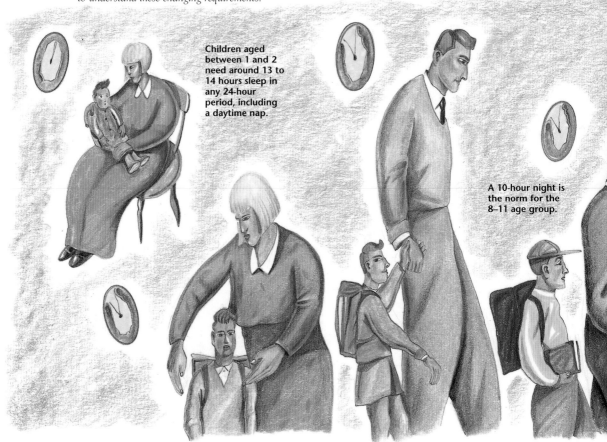

Children aged between 1 and 2 need around 13 to 14 hours sleep in any 24-hour period, including a daytime nap.

A 10-hour night is the norm for the 8–11 age group.

By 3 or 4, most children drop their daytime nap, but still need around 12 hours sleep a night.

Children need 10 or 11 hours sleep a night by the time they reach 5 or 6 years of age.

long winter period, many young children find the going hard and occasionally succumb to excessive tiredness and illness.

Teenage Sleep Times

Body growth is phenomenal during the first year after birth, when sleep needs are extensive. Between the ages of 3 and 10, growth is slow but steady, and sleep demands are influenced by activity as much as by growth. At puberty, there is again an enormous acceleration in growth, which continues until adult size is reached. Deep, slow-wave sleep is necessary for the secretion of the pubertal and growth hormones needed for development, and sleep patterns reflect this. Most noticeable, perhaps, is the teenager's reluctance to get up in the mornings. This is partly related to the time

he or she went to bed, but is also linked to the shift in the late sleep phase created by greater deep sleep needs.

Given the opportunity to sleep as much as necessary, most adolescents would average about nine hours. Many manage on less, but they build up a sleep deficit. At weekends they tend to sleep much later, often until noon, which distorts their sleep cycle quite dramatically. Circadian rhythms are affected, and the sleep/wake cycle becomes delayed. This results in difficulty waking in the morning, and being less alert at the beginning of the school day. The only solution is to shift the going-to-sleep time back progressively by 15 minutes a day, toward a more realistic one, while insisting on waking at a consistent hour every morning. It takes time to rearrange the pattern – but can be done.

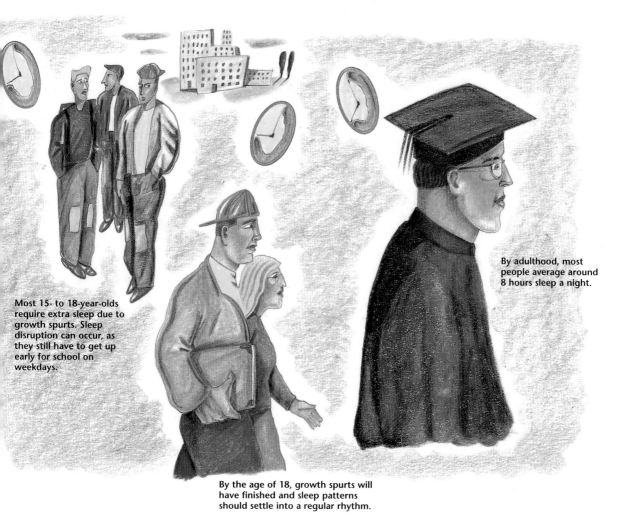

Most 15- to 18-year-olds require extra sleep due to growth spurts. Sleep disruption can occur, as they still have to get up early for school on weekdays.

By adulthood, most people average around 8 hours sleep a night.

By the age of 18, growth spurts will have finished and sleep patterns should settle into a regular rhythm.

Pregnancy

During the first three months of pregnancy, fatigue is considered a normal symptom. This is thought to be related to alterations in hormonal secretions: the increase in progesterone, the presence of human chorionic growth hormone, and the effects of these on the production of cortisol, adrenalin, and other hormones that can affect the sleep/wake cycle. The impact on sleep needs should reduce between 14 and 16 weeks of pregnancy, as the placenta becomes operational and hormonal activity settles down.

In addition, the fetus is growing at an extraordinary rate during the first few months. The growth requirements of the developing baby place a physical demand on the mother's body, and there is an increased need for sleep. To be sure that in meeting your baby's needs you don't neglect your own, a nutritious diet is especially important (see pages 70–71). Iron-deficiency anemia will leave an expectant mother feeling listless, so try increasing your intake of iron-rich foods, such as red meat, dark green vegetables, and apricots, before resorting to iron supplements.

Sleep Serene

Later on, tiredness can also derive from the physical demand of carrying extra weight. As the abdomen swells, getting comfortable in bed can be difficult. If you have always slept on your stomach, it will take time to adapt to sleeping on your side. Sleeping on your back can also become increasingly uncomfortable as the weight of the growing baby compresses

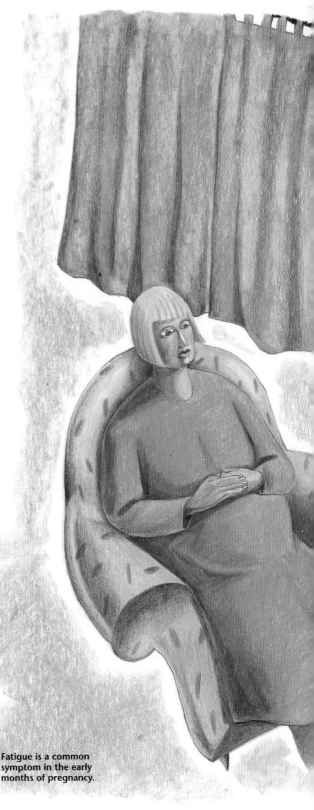

Fatigue is a common symptom in the early months of pregnancy.

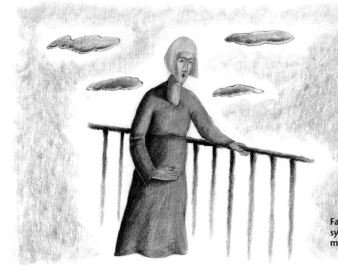

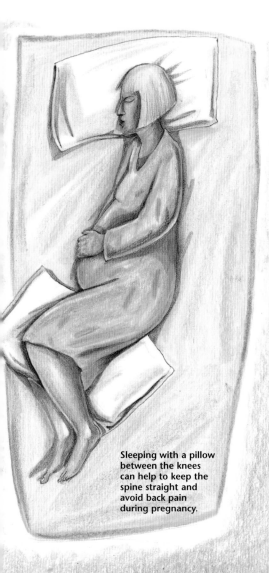

Sleeping with a pillow between the knees can help to keep the spine straight and avoid back pain during pregnancy.

During the later months of pregnancy, the stress of carrying around the increased body weight can cause tiredness.

other organs. Sleeping in a semi-recumbent position can be more comfortable – and ease heartburn. Lying on your side with a small pillow between your legs to avoid twisting your spine, or tucking a pillow under the weight of the abdomen, can help but no solution can equal the bliss of that first proper sleep after the baby is born, when your body feels like your own again.

Anxiety about becoming a mother, or the impending birth, can make sleep elusive if you switch into worry mode at bedtime or around 4 a.m. A number of relaxation and stress-reducing steps (see pages 82–83) can be helpful, and certain herbal remedies (see pages 102–103) can also be useful.

Adjustments After the Birth

After the birth, sleep can be a longed-for but elusive commodity, as you adjust to infant demands and new parenthood. Milk production and breastfeeding use up a lot of maternal energy, and sleep should be as plentiful as possible in the early days. You will be amazed at how little sleep you can manage on, but when you get some time for yourself and it's a choice between dusting the living room and grabbing forty winks – take the nap every time!

◀ *In the early weeks of pregnancy, exhaustion is the result of increased hormonal activity. Toward the end of pregnancy, it's the result of coping with additional body weight. Sleeping with a pillow between the knees can help, but nothing can compare to that first good night's sleep after the baby is born.*

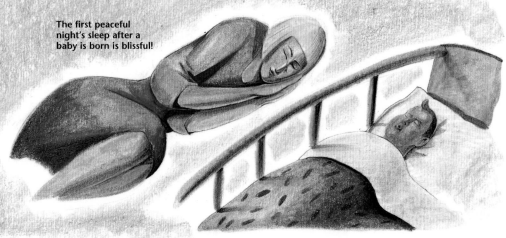

The first peaceful night's sleep after a baby is born is blissful!

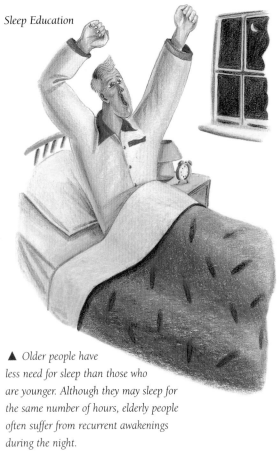

▲ *Older people have less need for sleep than those who are younger. Although they may sleep for the same number of hours, elderly people often suffer from recurrent awakenings during the night.*

Illness and Getting Older

Whether you are 2, 22, or 82, when you are sick your body needs to rest and recuperate. During sickness and convalescence, it is not unusual to sleep for long periods day and night, according to the severity of the condition. However, illness itself can make sleep difficult. Disturbed breathing, an irritating cough, fever, and pain can all interfere. Wherever possible, symptoms should be alleviated to aid sleep, with medical help if necessary.

The Influence of SAD

Seasonal Affective Disorder (SAD) – or winter depression, as it is sometimes termed – seems to alter sleep patterns in susceptible people, making insomnia more likely. If sleeplessness tends to affect you most in winter, light therapy may provide a solution. It involves sitting in front of a specially constructed "light box," which provides full-spectrum light for a prescribed number of hours each day. It can improve sleep patterns by creating the conditions in which waking up and daytime hormones function effectively. It can also counteract the dominance of melatonin production from the pineal gland that can arise from lack of light.

Depression and Stress

Psychological illness can cause severe problems with sleep. Insomnia, and in particular early morning waking without

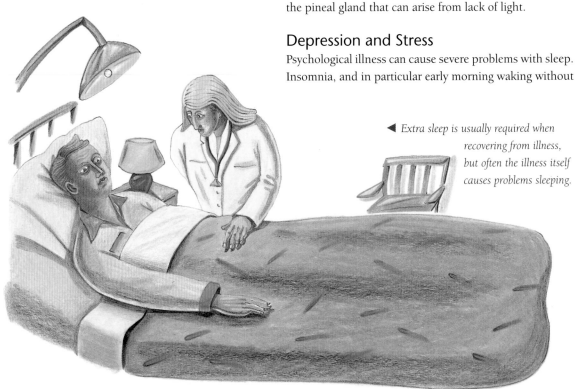

◀ *Extra sleep is usually required when recovering from illness, but often the illness itself causes problems sleeping.*

being able to return to sleep, is a classic symptom of depression. Stress can cause partial arousals during sleep; these contribute to daytime tiredness which, in turn, increases stress. Sleep apnea (see pages 42–43) can be a factor in reducing levels of oxygen to the brain, which can sometimes result in personality changes. Always consult your doctor when sleep problems persist – whether or not you can see a reason for them. Accurate diagnosis can lead you to the most suitable self-help steps, in conjunction with some short-term medication, if necessary.

Age-related Problems

As we age, our physical need for sleep, and in particular deep, slow-wave sleep, is reduced. Although the length of time spent asleep may remain fairly constant, sleep is lighter, with more awakenings. Women tend to suffer more than men with sleep problems, and may find that the menopause disrupts their sleep. Many women complain of being awoken by hot flashes and sweating but laboratory-based research showed that the beginnings of an awakening usually preceded the hot flash. However, this rise in body temperature, at an inappropriate time in the sleep cycle, disrupts sleep considerably. Hormone replacement therapy may help some women, but there are self-help remedies that you can use to alleviate menopausal symptoms that disturb your sleep. One recommendation is to take a combination of vitamin E, selenium, and vitamin C with bioflavonoids.

Sleep problems can also be complicated by age-onset illnesses, such as arthritis, which cause intermittent pain during sleep. Diminished physical activity and less exposure to daylight can also create difficulties with sleep in an older person. Reduced intellectual stimulation and the resultant boredom sometimes mean napping intermittently during the day, which further disrupts nighttime sleep. There is also some evidence that circadian rhythms (see pages 36–37) become desynchronized in certain elderly people, disturbing their sleep/wake patterns. Nighttime wakefulness is stressful, and if it is complicated by physical illness – a chest or other infection, for example – it can cause distressing symptoms of confusion.

Improvements in sleep hygiene (see pages 20–29) are the best way to tackle sleep problems associated with aging. They cannot solve all the difficulties, but they can certainly bring about improvements.

▼ *Young adults need the regenerating benefits of deep sleep, and reach deep-sleep stages several times during the night.*

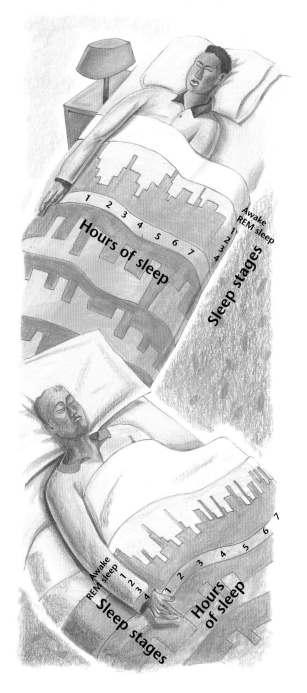

▲ *Our sleep patterns change as we age, with less need for the deeper, more restorative stages of sleep.*

Traveling

Any disruption to your routine can affect your sleep patterns. This happens most obviously when you travel, particularly if you cross time zones. A similar effect occurs as a result of shift work; chopping and changing your time on and off requires continual adjustment to match the social patterns of other people. When traveling you add the distorting effect of sleeping in a strange environment, away from the "clues" you associate with your personal sleep habits.

A strange bed, unfamiliar surroundings, different food, and unaccustomed noises can all contribute to disturbed sleep. On a business trip this could have a major impact on your performance, whereas on vacation you are less likely to be concerned. If you have also traveled across a number of time zones, being out of sync with your body clock will affect the way you feel, and your functioning can be considerably impaired.

Jet Lag

The circadian rhythms, on which your sleeping and waking are based (see pages 36–37), are well able to adjust – but this takes time. In the course of adapting to new patterns you will be at odds with your internal timing for temperature variations, hormone secretions, feelings of hunger, and other bodily functions, including the timing of sleepiness and alertness. This is what we understand as jet lag.

Retraining your circadian rhythms is easier if you are exposed to more rather than less light. So traveling west, which lengthens the number of daylight hours you experience, is easier than traveling east. For example, flying from Los Angeles to London will cause a more difficult adjustment than traveling back. The eight-hour time difference will, on the journey back to Los Angeles, take about two days to accommodate, while the outward journey from L.A. to London can take up to a week to readjust fully.

Taking Melatonin

Because of its natural role in defining the body's sleep/wake pattern, melatonin (see pages 36–37) is sometimes used by travelers to help retrain their circadian rhythms. It is most effective in treating the sleep-onset insomnia that can arise after traveling from west to east, and works relatively well provided you get up at the new morning time to maximize daylight hours. If you use melatonin, do not drive, operate machinery, or attempt to perform tasks requiring alertness for four to five hours after taking it. This rules out its suitability for shift workers, although it might be appropriate, with

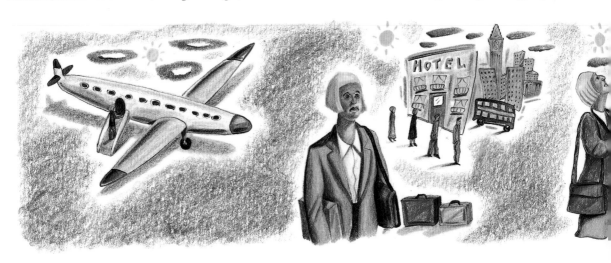

Jet lag is worse if you travel from west to east. If you leave Los Angeles at midday and fly to London, for example, when you reach your destination your body clock will think it's time to sleep.

Unfortunately, the new time zone is eight hours ahead and everyone else at your destination will soon be waking, ready for a new day. It is best to follow the new time structure as soon as possible.

On the outward journey from west to east, when you will be losing daylight hours, it can take up to a week for your circadian rhythms to adjust fully before you can begin to enjoy your vacation to the full.

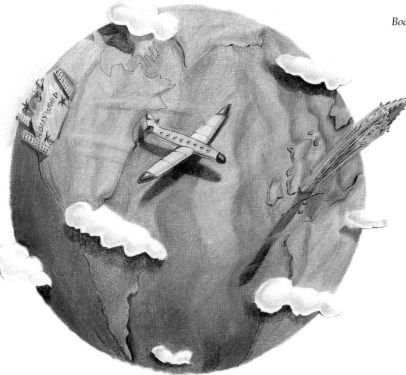

Traveling Tips

• Operate within the new time structure as soon as you can – even on the flight if possible, but certainly on arrival. This will give your body clock better clues on which to base its adjustment. Try to eat, sleep, and get up in keeping with local times.

• Try to get adequate rest in the days immediately prior to a long trip, so that you are not feeling exhausted before you start. This improves your chances of adjustment.

• Do not overindulge in alcohol during the flight. It tends to dehydrate the body, especially at high altitudes, and cause sleep disruptions. If you arrive during daylight hours and feel exhausted, take only a short nap to recuperate.

• Avoid sleeping excessively during the adjustment period.

• Use earplugs to shut out any noise disturbance to which you are excessively sensitive.

the proper precautions, in the initial adaptation period for those working night shifts permanently. It is readily available in the U.S. and sold through health food stores in numerous other countries, but it was recently banned from health stores in the U.K., where a synthetic but identical compound is available on prescription.

▲ ▼ *Traveling across time zones disrupts the body's circadian rhythms. This disruption is known as jet lag.*

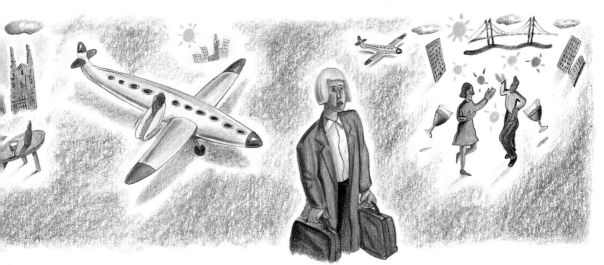

The return journey, from east to west, will also affect your circadian rhythms. If you leave London at midday, by the time you arrive back in Los Angeles, your body clock will again tell you it's almost time for bed.

Unfortunately, due to the time difference, everyone else will still be fully awake, enjoying the day your body clock thinks is over! This time, however, with an increase in daylight hours, it should only take around two days for your circadian rhythms to adjust.

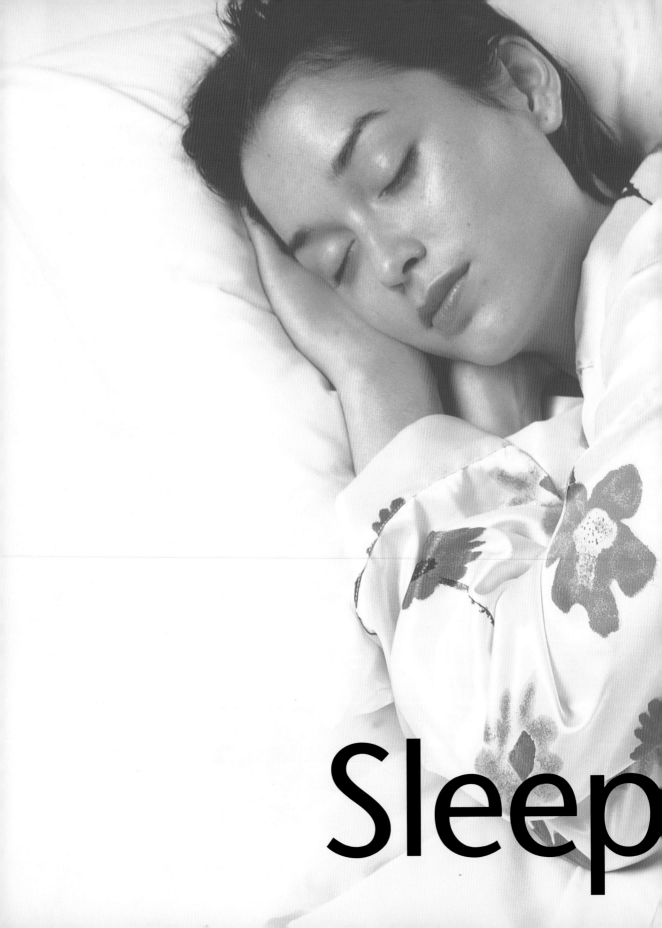

Sleep

Persistent sleep disorder is often symptomatic of other lifestyle problems. For example, your daily level of stress may be disrupting your ability to relax, rest, and sleep well. The balance of your life may be out of kilter, or a single source of upset, such as a bereavement or a job change, may have thrown your system off course. If this is the case, you need to approach your sleep disturbance holistically – as a symptom to be relieved by addressing the problem in its entirety.

Solutions

Therapies for Healthy Sleep

To cope with everything that life throws at us, we need to be in the best possible physical and emotional health. Sleep is an important part of this, and establishing good sleep habits benefits other aspects of life.

Chronic over-fatigue challenges the body's systems: tired muscles are more prone to strain; a continual sleep deficit can burden the immune system, making us more vulnerable to every passing bug; and persistent tiredness increases the risk of accidental injury as we lose our acuity and dexterity. The busier our lives become, the more we tend to neglect our sleep needs, overlooking the importance of sleep in enabling the body to utilize its restorative functions.

Lifestyle changes are not always easy, and you may need to devote some time to discovering which changes are more beneficial, and which additional aids, such as alternative or complementary therapies, are helpful. Some treatments are specifically directed at sleep problems – a herbal remedy, for example – while others are more holistically beneficial. In the case of feng shui this would include the harmonious arrangement of the environment where you plan to sleep. There are also many straightforward ways to boost our general health and well-being through diet and levels of regular enjoyable exercise.

There may well remain occasions when sleep is elusive, and some of us are more prone to this than others. But if

◀ *Stress is a common cause of sleeplessness, and most people find relaxation techniques and stretching exercises extremely beneficial.*

▼ *It is important for each individual to find those remedies, or a therapist, that work for them. Passionflower is often prescribed by herbalists for insomnia.*

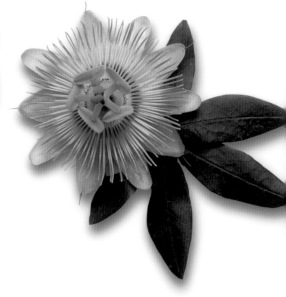

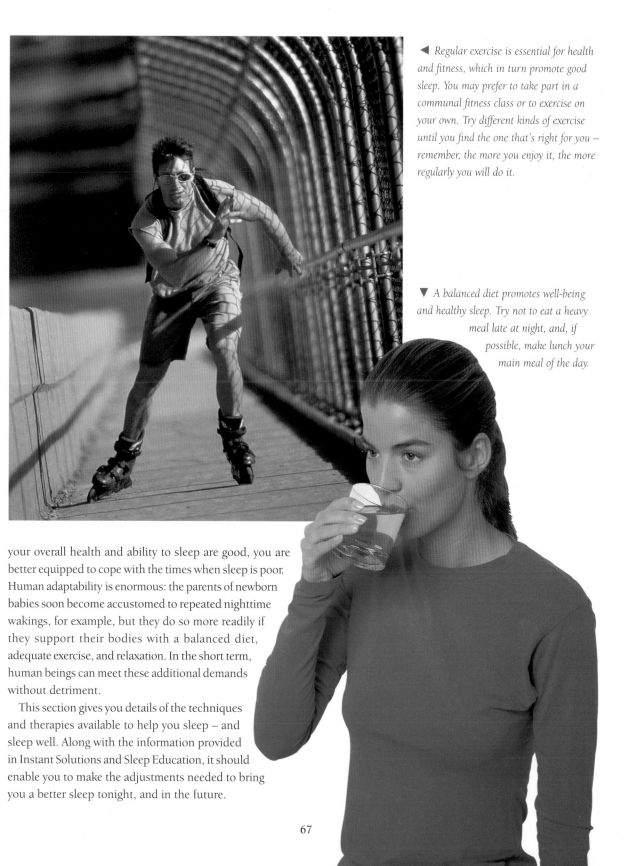

◀ *Regular exercise is essential for health and fitness, which in turn promote good sleep. You may prefer to take part in a communal fitness class or to exercise on your own. Try different kinds of exercise until you find the one that's right for you – remember, the more you enjoy it, the more regularly you will do it.*

▼ *A balanced diet promotes well-being and healthy sleep. Try not to eat a heavy meal late at night, and, if possible, make lunch your main meal of the day.*

your overall health and ability to sleep are good, you are better equipped to cope with the times when sleep is poor. Human adaptability is enormous: the parents of newborn babies soon become accustomed to repeated nighttime wakings, for example, but they do so more readily if they support their bodies with a balanced diet, adequate exercise, and relaxation. In the short term, human beings can meet these additional demands without detriment.

This section gives you details of the techniques and therapies available to help you sleep – and sleep well. Along with the information provided in Instant Solutions and Sleep Education, it should enable you to make the adjustments needed to bring you a better sleep tonight, and in the future.

Assessing Your Problem

You know you feel tired, or you know you have trouble getting to sleep, but you're not sure what's causing your particular sleep problem. The Crisis Management Plan on pages 12–19 will help you to improve things immediately, but in order to find a long-term solution, you need to discover the cause of your sleep problem, and this may take a little time.

To discover the underlying causes of your sleep problem, it is a good idea to keep a sleep diary, like the one shown below. It may take a little time before a pattern emerges, but once it does, it will be helpful in finding a long-term solution. And if you feel it necessary to consult a doctor at some point about your sleeping problems, the information in this sleep diary will be helpful to him or her in reaching a diagnosis and planning an appropriate course of action.

By keeping a sleep diary, the cause of your problem may become immediately apparent: night waking caused by too much alcohol late at night, on a regular basis; or perhaps insomnia caused by working too hard and not getting enough physical exercise or relaxation; or even a chronic insufficient sleep syndrome from consistently going to bed at too late an hour, for example. Most of us can discover the main causes of our poor sleep fairly quickly, but tackling a sleep problem,

SLEEP DIARY	Day 1	Day 2	Day 3	Day 4
Time awoke?				
Woken by alarm or not?				
Any periods of sleepiness or naps taken during the day?				
Daytime activity – work, time off, etc?				
Any exercise taken? What form? For how long? When?				
Any physical ailments or illnesses?				
Any caffeine taken? How much? When?				
Any alcohol drunk? How much? When?				
Any medication taken? What? When?				
Time of last meal eaten?				
Time went to bed?				
Time fell asleep?				
Times awake during the night? At what time? For how long?				
Snoring? Breathing disruptions?				

in a way that is appropriate to you, may take some time before it is fully effective. An uncomfortable bed is relatively easy to solve, but if your problem is sleep apnea caused by obesity, for example, it will take time to lose sufficient weight to alleviate the problem.

In addition, the fear of being unable to sleep may take longer to diminish than the reasons the inability to sleep arose in the first place. Many people feel an onset of panic when they go to bed, believing that sleep will elude them, and it takes time to become confident that new sleep habits can really be effective, especially if they don't appear to work at first. This is an additional benefit of the sleep diary – it can be used to monitor sleep improvements as well as sleep problems, and to provide you with tangible proof that a therapy is working and that the problem is soluble.

Many approaches and possible solutions to sleep problems are discussed in this section. If you tried them all, there wouldn't be time left for sleep! So you need to plan a course of action, as a follow-up to the Crisis Management Plan, to suit your individual needs. This will require a certain amount of honesty about what lifestyle changes are essential, and a firm commitment to making them. If a heavy meal late at night means regularly waking up with indigestion at 2 a.m., then this will have to change – no matter how much you enjoy late-night dining! Map out a schedule, like the one shown below, and try to follow it over a period of a couple of weeks to see what is, and what isn't, working. Once your schedule is firmly established and working, it will be possible to introduce some flexibility – a supper party once in a while won't hurt, because you will know what to do to avoid any resulting sleep disruption from becoming a problem again.

In reorganizing a daytime schedule to help promote better sleep patterns, bear in mind that your overall aim is to rebalance your life – sleep should be a sustaining part of your life, but you shouldn't rely on sleep alone to restore you. A balanced life should include each of the following in some degree: exercise and relaxation; doing something for yourself; doing something with other people; having fun; and time for some sort of spiritual reflection. Any schedule you devise for yourself should pay attention to these areas as well as to sleep itself.

Day 5	Day 6	Day 7

Sample Schedule

- Wake at 7.30 a.m., even at weekends
- Practice meditation for 10 minutes
- Lunchtime swim three times a week
- No coffee after 3 p.m.
- Weekly massage and osteopathic treatment for neck and back pain
- Eat no later than 7 p.m., and drink only one glass of wine with the meal
- No work after 9 p.m.
- No television after 10 p.m.
- Warm candlelit bath with lavender oil added
- Milky drink and soft music in bed
- Read for a while
- Switch off lights by 11 p.m. at the latest

Diet

Most people know that their bodies require an adequate intake of different kinds of foods in order to remain healthy, and that their diet should provide a balanced amount of carbohydrates, protein, fats, vitamins, and minerals. The simplest way to consider your diet is to divide food into four groups, bearing in mind that different foods can provide similar nutrients, but some foods provide them in a higher concentration than others.

• Carbohydrates include a range of foods, such as potatoes, breads, wholemeal cereals, pasta, and rice. They are usually low in fats and contain a certain amount of protein, vitamins, and minerals. Some carbohydrates, such as brown rice and wholewheat pasta, are known as "complex carbohydrates," because they take longer to break down into the simple sugars that cells need for energy, so providing a slower but more continuous energy source.

• **Fruits and vegetables** are the best providers of vitamins and minerals, especially when eaten fresh. They also supply fiber, which contributes bulk and enables the digestive system to function properly.

• **Dairy foods**, such as milk, cheese, and yogurt, are a good source of calcium, protein, and B vitamins, and full-fat or fortified dairy products contain the fat-soluble vitamins A and D.

• **Protein suppliers** include meat, fish, eggs, pulses, and nuts. They also contain some minerals, and vitamins from the B group.

▶ *Ensuring a balanced daily intake of food – carbohydrates, fruits, vegetables, diary products, and protein – can help improve sleep.*

A point to check, and change if necessary, is your intake of fat and refined sugar, which are often introduced during the cooking or processing of foods. Steaming or broiling (grilling) food is more nutritious than boiling or frying, and fresh foods are healthier than processed ones. The old saying "Take breakfast like a king, lunch like a prince, and supper like a pauper" is a wise one, although not always easy to follow. A substantial breakfast, with an adequate supply of complex carbohydrates, is an excellent start to the day. A light meal in the evening is better than going to bed on an over-full stomach, which could lead to indigestion and sleep disturbances. It is important to eat enough food prior to sleep, however, so that your night is not disrupted by hunger pangs. If you complete your last main meal more than four hours before bedtime, have a last snack, consisting of a milky drink and some carbohydrate – a wholemeal sandwich or a bowl of cereal, perhaps – up to an hour before you go to bed.

Whatever your level of physical activity, your body expends up to 70 percent of its energy every day just maintaining cells, building new tissue, and keeping body systems and organs working. Although our energy needs vary during our lives – a growing teenager has greater energy demands than an elderly person, for example – these can be met by adjusting the calorific value of the foods we eat. The teenager would benefit from the extra calories available in whole, or full-fat, milk, while the elderly person could manage satisfactorily on skimmed or semi-skimmed milk.

Food and sleep are essential components of a healthy life, and both contribute greatly to the body's ability to function efficiently and restore itself. Eating nutritiously combined with adequate amounts of regular, restful sleep will ensure that the body can work efficiently and resist illness.

A Balanced Diet

Nutritionists generally agree that a balanced daily diet can be neatly encapsulated in the formula "12345+."
one serving of meat or meat equivalent;
two servings of dairy products;
three servings of fruit;
four servings of vegetables;
five servings of bread, cereals, pasta, or rice;
+ a little of what you fancy!

Obviously proportions can vary slightly on some days, but this is a good general guide.

71

Exercise

Expending energy can increase tiredness, but regular exercise brings additional benefits. Physical activity is one way of reducing muscle tension. If you sit in an office all day, working on a computer, one set of muscles is used repetitively while others do not move at all. The resulting muscular tension can be exacerbated by flopping in front of the television in order to relax. The musculo-skeletal strain can make it increasingly difficult to relax the muscles as a precursor to sleep. At its worst, muscle tension causes pain that prevents restful sleep.

▶ *Our bodies need adequate physical activity each day to function well, and this can help improve sleep. Badminton, tennis, golf, swimming, and walking are just some of the activities you can do.*

Exercise also promotes healthy breathing. At rest, we tend to breathe in a relatively shallow way, which can become shallower still during periods of stress and tension. This can escalate until rapid breathing, using only the upper chest, contributes to a feeling of suffocation. It is possible to learn to breathe more deeply (see pages 84–85), but regular exercise encourages this to happen naturally. The increased oxygen intake is beneficial to all of the body cells, and makes you feel both more alert and more relaxed.

A recent study by the Health Education Authority in the UK showed that 60 percent of men and 70 percent of women are insufficiently active to benefit their health. According to a national survey in 1992, 50 percent of women over the age of 50 did not have enough leg power to climb stairs easily. But the good news from another piece of medical research was that gentle exercise for at least 3 hours a week improved muscle strength by 25 percent after only 12 weeks. So exercise is a must for health as well as sleep benefits. Choose physical activities that you enjoy and are therefore more likely to pursue regularly. It is best to aim for a combination of different activities. For example, swim twice a week, take a twenty-minute walk five days a week (perhaps by walking to work or to school), and spend five minutes every night doing stretching exercises.

It is useful to create a balance between aerobic exercise and stretching exercises – contrasting jogging with yoga, for example. As with everything else, balancing your needs is a positive way to approach exercise. If you have a particular health requirement, seek the advice of a physiotherapist or physical therapist about what particular kind of exercise will be the most beneficial for you.

Many people find that minor aches and pains tolerated for years diminish when they adopt a regular routine of gentle exercise. Circulation improves, joint pain lessens, muscular tension decreases, stamina improves, and feelings of alertness and well-being are enhanced. And that is in addition to the reduced risk of heart disease and strokes, the prevention of osteoporosis, the lessening of depression, and improvement to diabetes. Whatever your situation or physical state, the right amount of exercise can only make you feel – and sleep – better.

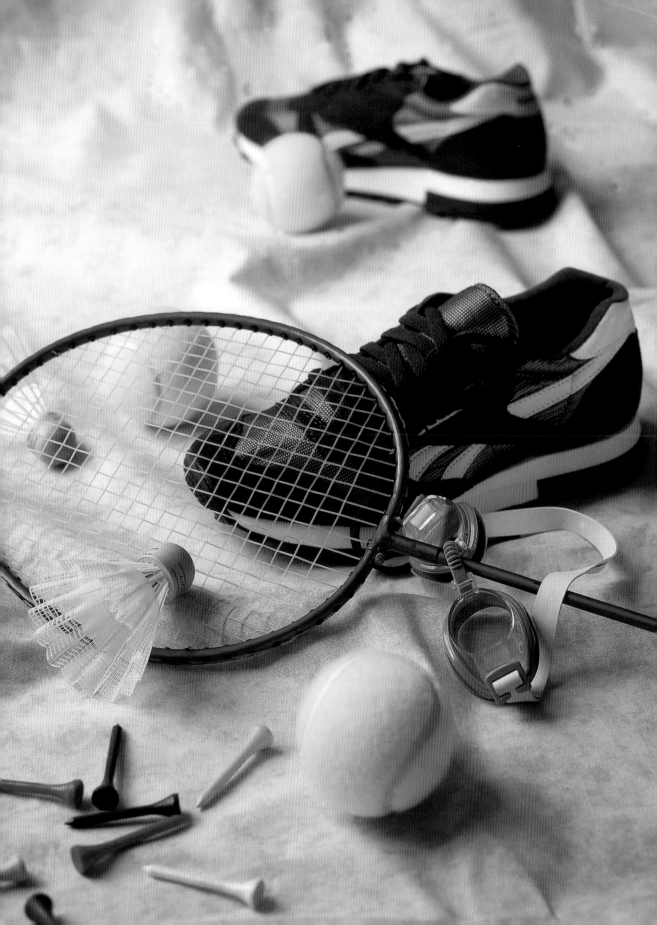

Yoga

The practice of yoga has existed in the East for at least 5000 years, but it was only introduced to the West in the 19th century. It became extremely popular in the 1960s, when those who discovered its benefits included the violinist Sir Yehudi Menuhin. His playing career was threatened by a frozen shoulder until he consulted a yoga teacher whose exercises relieved the problem.

The word yoga comes from the Sanskrit, meaning union, and the primary aim of yoga practice is to create a union, or balance, between body and mind. This is achieved through the postures, or *asanas*, combined with the breathing exercises, or *pranayamas*. The idea behind *prana* is similar to the Chinese concept of *qi*. In the theory of acupuncture, the body's *qi*, or energy, flows along invisible channels known as meridians, whereas in yoga the *prana* flows along *nadis*: poor health is thought to occur when there is a blockage in these channels.

Yoga practice is designed to stimulate the seven major *chakras*, the points of focused energy in the body, which have both positive and negative qualities. The *chakras* are found at the crown of the head, the center of the forehead, the throat, the solar plexus, the spine, the heart, and the navel. There are about 80 main yoga postures, although only around 20 are used regularly. For each *asana* there is a counter *asana*, which balances the physical effects of the posture.

Yoga undoubtedly aids relaxation and reduces stress, so it can be extremely beneficial for those who find sleeping difficult. Studies have shown that yoga has a part to play in the active management of conditions such as asthma, high blood pressure, back pain, mild cases of non-insulin-dependent diabetes, and chronic anxiety. Research published by the Yoga Biomedical Trust in the 1980s showed that among 542 sufferers from chronic insomnia, 82 percent found that yoga had helped them.

► *This yoga sequence, the "Mountain Breath," promotes healthy breathing. Stand with your arms by your sides and breathe out slowly (1). Then breathe in slowly, raising your arms out to the side (2). Continue until your arms are fully stretched above your head (3). Link your thumbs and hold the air in your lungs for a few seconds. Breathe out and lower your arms. Repeat five times a day.*

To learn yoga initially, you need the guidance of a skilled teacher. Although practicing at home usually becomes routine, you can continue to benefit from regular supervision, and the opportunity to extend yoga techniques. Classes generally begin with a warm-up of stretching exercises, followed by a sequence of *asanas* alternating with breathing exercises, and culminate with the best-known relaxation pose, the *savasana* or "Corpse" pose. Some yoga classes include the teaching of meditation, known as *samayama*.

Yoga is suitable for most ages and abilities, and a good teacher will check with each individual in his or her class for any physical problem that could make certain postures difficult or damaging. The yoga most widely practiced in the West is *Hatha* yoga. *Ha* means sun, and *tha* means moon, so together they represent the joining of the sun and moon: the union of the male and female aspects of an individual, and the union or balancing of the body and mind. The focus is on postures, breathing, and meditation, although the actual practice depends on both student and teacher.

One of the many benefits of learning yoga is that the postures can be used at any time to alleviate stress and promote relaxation. People who practice yoga often use a series of postures before bed to stretch and relax muscles, relieve tension, and so promote sleep. Similarly, they begin the day with a sequence of stretching exercises, the most famous being the "Salute to the Sun."

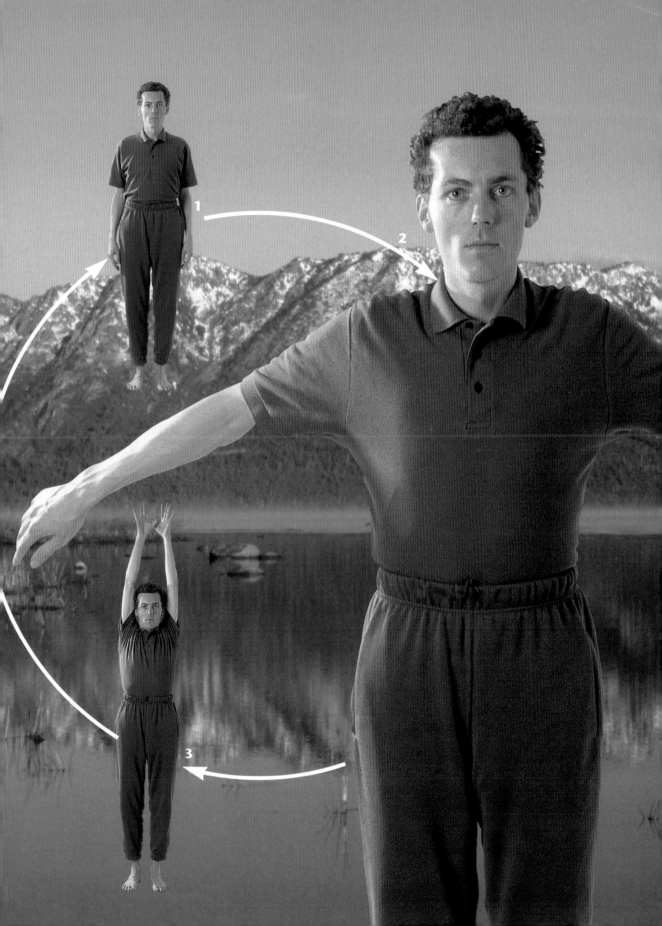

Tai Chi

Tai chi developed from the martial art of kung fu, but was devised as a non-competitive antidote to the more aggressive martial arts. Its full name is *t'ai chi chuan*. *T'ai chi* means "the supreme unity," and *chuan* means the "fist" or "container." The focus of tai chi is to balance the two complementary energy forces of *yin* and *yang* within the body, stabilizing and harmonizing their fluctuations to restore health and well-being.

▶ *Tai chi can benefit all age groups and promote a more tranquil approach to life. It consists of basic postures, which are linked into a single, flowing movement. The postures shown here, clockwise from bottom left, are: push, press, lifting hands, golden rooster, kick with heel, seven stars, sweep lotus, and shoulder stroke (center).*

As with other Eastern philosophies, the principle of good health in tai chi rests on the fundamental concept that mind and body must be in harmony with each other; the body cannot work proficiently if it is inhibited by anxiety, tension, fear, or irritability. Practices such as tai chi, although physical, center on the interplay between the body and the mind. As one calms the other, the effect is completed and good health is restored.

The slow, graceful movements of tai chi make them suitable for all ages and physical abilities. Although not an aerobic form of exercise, it is physical exercise nonetheless; it enhances suppleness and flexibility, and can therefore ease many joint and muscular pains. Because it improves posture, it can also combat the aches and pains that come from the sedentary lifestyle that many of us lead. The unhurried movements of tai chi, which are precise but fluid, are the antithesis of the way in which most of us conduct our lives, and can do a lot to counteract the detrimental effects of our everyday routines on our ability to unwind and to sleep well.

You will need to join a class to learn tai chi, so that you can see and copy the movements accurately. Although it can take between three months and two years to become proficient in tai chi, with a good teacher and plenty of practice, the benefits can become apparent very quickly.

Qigong

Similar in form to tai chi, qigong is a series of exercises designed to stimulate the *qi* or *chi* – the body's intrinsic energy.

Qigong is a component of traditional Chinese medicine, along with herbalism and acupuncture, and means "energy cultivation." Through exercises that focus on breathing, posture, and visualization, qigong aims to unblock, stimulate, and strengthen the internal flow of the body's *qi*.

Qigong is sometimes referred to as "meditation in motion," because of its combination of visualization techniques and breathing exercises with gentle, flowing movements. For those who find conventional approaches to meditation difficult, qigong can be a useful means of focusing the mind and calming the body. Like tai chi, its slow and graceful poses contribute to physical well-being as well as mental relaxation. Studies in China have reported its efficacy in relieving symptoms of insomnia, depression, anxiety, arthritis, and pain.

Expert tuition is required to learn qigong, but it is easy to continue practicing it alone.

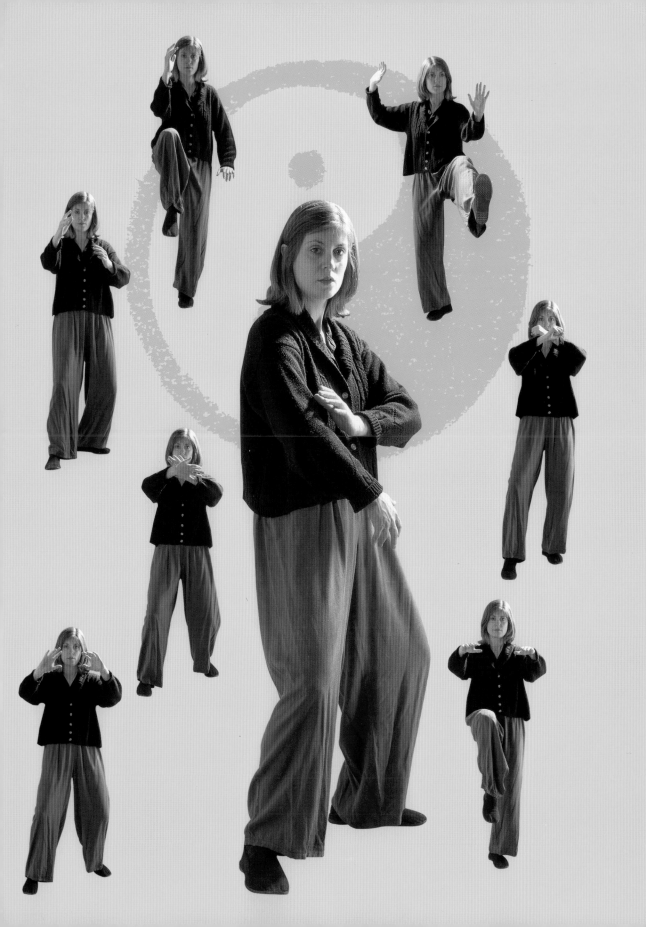

Massage

Touch is possibly the first sense our bodies experience as we develop in the uterus, and healthy childhood development is partly dependent on the benefits of positive touch. Children who are regularly cuddled and physically cherished grow better, generally flourish, and are less susceptible to disease. They tend to be more outgoing and happy – and, significantly, they sleep better. In adult life, touch can bring similar benefits, and invokes fundamental feelings of love and security.

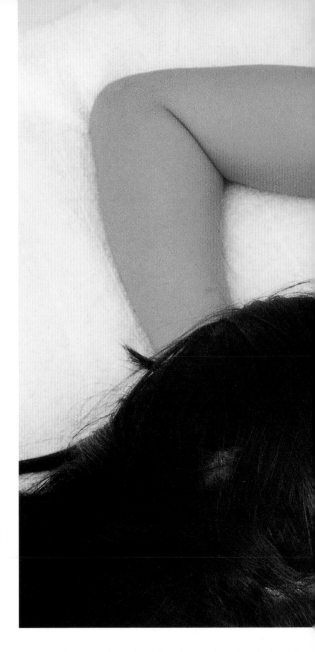

Massage can relieve the muscular tension and feelings of stress that build up during the day. It is used therapeutically in sports clinics and health centers to smooth knots in connective tissue and muscle fascia caused by injury or tension, to improve circulation, tone muscles, and generally invigorate the body. Some forms of Thai massage, the deep-tissue Indian *marma* massage, and the Chinese *tuina* are all specifically designed to tackle deep-seated muscular problems. Such forms of massage can be beneficial where physical discomfort is contributing to a sleep problem, but the gentle, relaxing massage designed as a precursor to sleep is different. It is therefore important to discuss the techniques and their aims before undertaking any massage treatment.

However, the usefulness of the right kind of massage in promoting relaxation and sleep is renowned. Physical touch both relaxes muscles and creates the feelings of security necessary in order to "let go" and fall asleep, an effect often witnessed by professional therapists. Fortunately, you can achieve the same results at home, either through self-massage techniques, or from a friend or partner. Better still, the more often you use massage this way, the more effective it becomes in treating sleep disorders. An additional benefit is that massage can soothe the giver as well as the receiver, and many couples find that it is a simple way of literally getting

back in touch with each other before the day's end. Learning a few basic techniques will improve the quality and enjoyment of your home massage. Include stroking, kneading, knuckling, static and circular pressure (using the thumbs), and percussion (a gentle drumming motion of the hands). Practice on a willing back to get an idea of the movements and how firmly to apply them, then move to different areas of the body, adapting your pressure as necessary. There are some areas of the body that you can massage on yourself; self-massage of your neck, abdomen, hands, arms, legs, and feet can be beneficial.

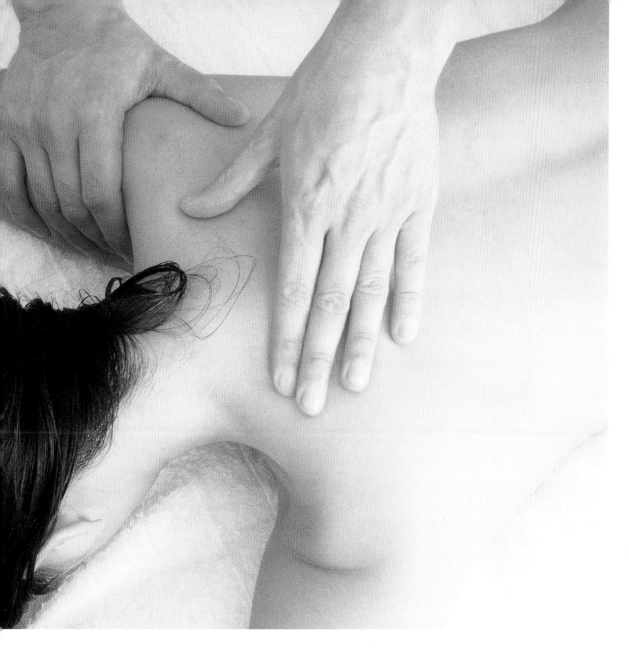

The environment in which you give or receive a massage should be private, comfortably warm, and quiet – such as your bedroom prior to sleep. Use oil to allow the hands to move freely over the body. This should be a vegetable- not a mineral-based oil, especially if you are massaging a baby or child, as their skins are very sensitive and a mineral-based oil could cause irritation. In fact, most baby oils are mineral-based, so they are not suitable for massaging babies at all. Almond oil is a good base to which you can add essential oils of your choice (see pages 80–81); olive oil could be too heavy and too pungent.

▲ *A back massage can help reduce muscle tension and pain, and promote restful sleep. Make sure the room is warm enough, and add a couple of drops of essential oil to the carrier oil, if liked. Pay special attention to muscles that feel tense and "knotted," a common occurrence at the base of the neck and shoulders, which can cause stress-related headaches. Vary the strokes used, and the pressure applied, to get the best results.*

Aromatherapy

The therapeutic use of essential oils, known as aromatherapy, is one of the fastest growing therapies in the Western world. The oils are produced by steam distillation from the flowers, leaves, bark, seeds, and even the fruit of plants. There are some 400 plant essences, with complex chemical structures, each possessing different characteristics and therapeutic values. For example, lavender has a calming effect, and sage is stimulating.

► *Essential oils can be added to bathwater, or to a carrier oil and used for massage. Alternatively, diluted oils can be vaporized, using a gentle heat source.*

The essential oils have a tiny molecular structure, which means that they can be absorbed through the skin into the bloodstream.

They can also enter the body through the nose. The smell of the oil stimulates an area of the brain known as the limbic system. This area is concerned with instinctive behavior, mood control, and emotions, and the link between human emotion and the release of certain body chemicals is well-known. Think how fear releases adrenalin, or how love releases endorphins, for example. So aromatherapy is believed to exercise effect on both physical and mental well-being.

Aromatherapy is recommended for stress-related conditions – particularly in combination with massage. Other ailments that respond well include digestive problems, some skin conditions, including eczema and rosacea, muscular aches and pains, period problems, and menopausal symptoms. British mental health organization, MIND, has reported that the use of aromatherapy by people with depression is particularly effective.

You can buy essential oils for yourself but guidance is needed to choose the most suitable, and certain cautions apply, so you should take advice from a qualified aromatherapist. Some essential oils should not be used during pregnancy, for example; these include basil, clary sage, myrrh, rosemary, sage, sweet marjoram, and thyme.

Essential oils are often recommended for sleep disorders and an aromatherapist can help you focus on the remedy that is right for you. If the cause of insomnia is depression, for example, it might be appropriate to treat the depression, with, say, neroli oil, which lifts the mood while calming the heart. If there is a need to encourage relaxation prior to sleep, adding lavender oil to a vaporizer in the bedroom may be helpful. Sometimes the associations of a particular smell can evoke a sense of peace and security. The warm, woody smell of sandalwood, added to the bathwater, may soothe and relax.

Essential oils can be used singly or in combination. An aromatherapist might mix a number of oils specifically for you. You can then utilize this blend at home in a variety of ways: through massage, vaporization, in the bath, or to scent a handkerchief or pillow.

Recommended Oils

The oils especially recommended for sleep problems include:

**Lavender Cypress
Rose Marjoram
Neroli Chamomile
Sandalwood Petitgrain**

Give yourself a face, neck, and shoulder massage, using two or three of the above oils – for example, lavender, neroli, and chamomile – combined in a sweet almond carrier oil. Then relax in a warm bath. The effects of the massage will be enhanced by the steamy inhalation of the aroma of the essential oils.

Dilutions

(per 2fl oz/50ml in each case)
Adults: 25 drops
Children over one year: 10 drops
Babies under one year: 5 drops
Halve the number of drops of oil if using on the face or neck.

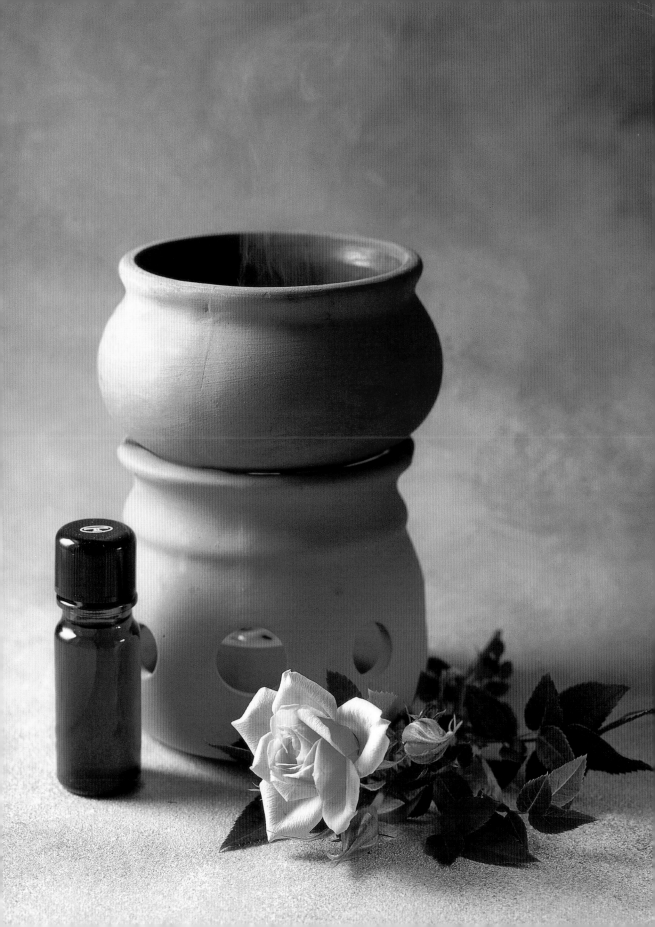

Relaxation

The art of relaxation is complex, and many people find it elusive. We feel as if it should come naturally, but for most of us it is a skill to be learned or relearned. Relaxation is not a passive activity, and it requires a combination of mental and physical skills to counteract the negative effects of too much stress and tension in our lives. It is worth making an effort to find the method of relaxation most suitable for you, because it makes everyday life more manageable, and falling asleep at night easier.

The first step we need to take toward achieving relaxation is to learn to feel the difference between muscle tension and muscle relaxation. Often when we think we are relaxed, we are in fact sitting with our jaw clamped tight or shoulders hunched, for example. Tension is priming our muscles for action. Living in this constant state of stimulation is physically exhausting, so if we relax, we actually conserve energy.

Exercise is one good way to aid relaxation. When you exercise your muscles, they are automatically tensed and released. Physical exertion also promotes deeper breathing, which increases the amount of oxygen taken into the body. By concentrating on the particular demands of a physical activity, the mind is often cleared of other thoughts for a period of time, thus promoting mental relaxation as well as physical release.

If you find mental relaxation difficult, focusing on physical relaxation first can help. A relaxed body promotes mental relaxation. Like most benefits, however, relaxation techniques must be practiced regularly to be effective. If this is an area you find hard, some guidance may be necessary. A number of therapists specialize in teaching self-help methods of relaxation, through specific exercises, or in conjunction with other therapies, such as massage, tai chi, or visualization, for example.

The benefits of learning how to relax are incalculable. It is a skill that you can practice anywhere to relieve stress and revitalize your body. And it could prove invaluable in inducing sleep when you go to bed or if you wake up during the night.

Relaxation Exercises

The following exercises will help you feel the difference between muscle tension and relaxation. Do them standing or sitting.

• Squeeze your hands into fists as tightly as possible and hold for a slow count of five; stretch the fingers for a slow count of five; then release and allow the hands to feel floppy.

• Stretch your arms high above your head and hold for a slow count of five; stretch the arms to the side to open up the chest, and hold for a slow count of five; then release and rest your forearms on your lap.

• With one hand resting loosely on the corresponding shoulder (right hand on right shoulder; left hand on left shoulder), rotate your elbow five times clockwise on a slow count of five, and then five times counter-clockwise. Repeat with the other arm.

• Raise your head to look up as far as you comfortably can; then look down; then move the head from one side to the other, before rotating your neck through a full circle to a slow count of five.

Drop your shoulders before each exercise, and be aware of their lowered position throughout. Keep the muscles of your lower abdomen soft, and breathe deeply into the abdomen on each slow count of five.

◀ *Physical tension often shows in the face. Ensure your facial muscles are relaxed, which will aid relaxation everywhere.*

Breathing Techniques

We all know how to breathe; we do it automatically all the time, to stay alive. However, many of us breathe inefficiently, using only the upper chest, as if we were about to take fright or flight. This encourages the body to remain in a constant state of alert, which continues through the night and can cause sleep disturbance.

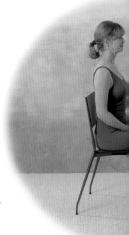

Stress can also affect breathing. In severe cases, panic attacks can cause hyperventilation and feelings of suffocation. Learning to breathe correctly, and acquiring breathing techniques for use in particular circumstances, can therefore be of enormous benefit. Proper breathing is also the key to successful relaxation and meditation. It involves using the diaphragm when breathing in and out. The diaphragm is the sheet of muscle that divides the chest from the abdomen. In moving up and down, it draws air into the lungs. By deliberately expanding the chest and using the diaphragm, you bring your breathing under conscious control, and you can then regularize and deepen it to contribute to relaxation.

Just as consciously tensing and relaxing your muscles promotes overall relaxation, so does consciously breathing deeply and slowly. When you feel stressed and "out of control," bringing your breathing back under control reduces panic. When you feel anxious, you tend instinctively to hold your breath, which restricts air intake and creates even greater tension. The result of everyday shallow breathing from the upper chest is also to limit the body's oxygen intake, which maintains an inappropriate level of arousal and increases feelings of negative fatigue. Once you acquire the habit of breathing correctly during the day, you will then be able to continue breathing correctly during the night, bringing the added benefit of deeper, more refreshing sleep.

Hyperventilation

Hyperventilation can cause anxiety, and be caused by it. Feeling panicky about an inability to sleep, combined with other anxieties, can affect breathing to the point of hyperventilation in susceptible people. Its effects can be alarming, but once its initial symptoms are controlled, it responds well to breathing techniques.

Hyperventilation describes excessively shallow and rapid breathing, using only the upper chest. This form of breathing eventually disturbs the oxygen/carbon dioxide ratio in the blood, causing tingling in the fingers, face, and feet. In severe cases, there may also be muscle pain and cramps. Hyperventilation is also associated with apnea (see pages 42–43), where breathing stops momentarily during sleep, as the body tries to normalize itself. This can be extremely distressing, frightening, and also self-perpetuating: anxiety causes the hyperventilation, which then increases the anxiety, and the fear over its occurrence and potential recurrence.

To deal with an attack, it helps to breathe in and out of a paper bag. To avoid an attack, practice breathing techniques on a regular basis, so that you can use them whenever it feels as if anxiety could escalate into hyperventilation.

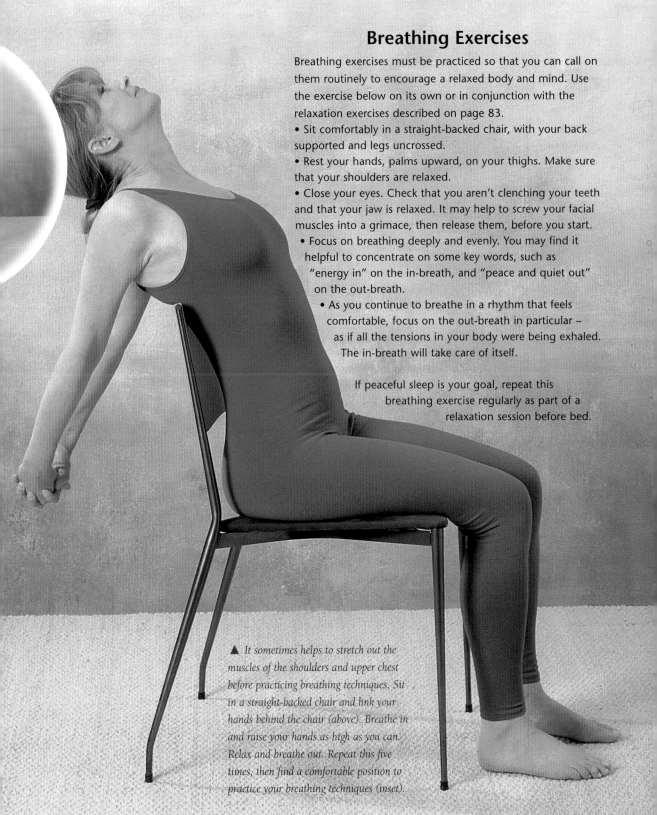

Breathing Exercises

Breathing exercises must be practiced so that you can call on them routinely to encourage a relaxed body and mind. Use the exercise below on its own or in conjunction with the relaxation exercises described on page 83.

• Sit comfortably in a straight-backed chair, with your back supported and legs uncrossed.

• Rest your hands, palms upward, on your thighs. Make sure that your shoulders are relaxed.

• Close your eyes. Check that you aren't clenching your teeth and that your jaw is relaxed. It may help to screw your facial muscles into a grimace, then release them, before you start.

• Focus on breathing deeply and evenly. You may find it helpful to concentrate on some key words, such as "energy in" on the in-breath, and "peace and quiet out" on the out-breath.

• As you continue to breathe in a rhythm that feels comfortable, focus on the out-breath in particular – as if all the tensions in your body were being exhaled. The in-breath will take care of itself.

If peaceful sleep is your goal, repeat this breathing exercise regularly as part of a relaxation session before bed.

▲ *It sometimes helps to stretch out the muscles of the shoulders and upper chest before practicing breathing techniques. Sit in a straight-backed chair and link your hands behind the chair (above). Breathe in and raise your hands as high as you can. Relax and breathe out. Repeat this five times, then find a comfortable position to practice your breathing techniques (inset).*

Meditation

Many of us find that what prevents sleep at night is a never-ending round of troublesome thoughts and worries. We feel that if only we could control these, sleep would be possible. But however hard we try to relax, and empty our minds, the minute our heads hit the pillow, it all begins again.

▶ *Whatever you choose to focus on when meditating, stick with it once you have started, as this will help your technique. A lighted candle is a good choice. Repeating a mantra, such as "om," the Sanskrit symbol of which is shown here, can also help.*

This is a situation where meditation can be wonderfully helpful. Like the relaxation and breathing exercises mentioned earlier, successful meditation takes regular practice, and it won't become fully effective immediately – although some of its benefits occur almost at once. Meditation can be self-taught, but the guidance of a teacher and joining a class provides support and will help you to develop the technique to a good level of proficiency.

Research has shown measurable benefits from regular meditation. During meditation, the pulse rate slows, blood pressure falls, blood supply to the body's extremities improves, and levels of stress hormones drop. Changes occur in brain-wave activity: there is a more rhythmical alpha wave pattern, found only in calm and relaxed states. This relaxation results in a feeling of refreshed alertness, although it can also be used to induce the calm needed before sleep.

Learning to Meditate

You need to practice for at least 10–15 minutes each day to become proficient at meditation. It is useful to set aside the same time each day, and to meditate in the same place, because then your body and mind begin to associate a particular set of circumstances with meditation.

Sit, rather than lie, in a position that will remain comfortable throughout. Use a chair or sit on the floor, but keep your back straight and supported. Rest your hands, palms upward, on your thighs, so that your arms are supported but your shoulders are relaxed. Close your eyes and begin focusing on your breathing. For the first few minutes, just concentrate on this. Then begin to deepen your breath, focusing on the out-breath. This is very similar to the breathing exercises described on page 85.

Continue to concentrate on keeping your breathing slow and steady, but at the same time, begin consciously to relax your body, starting with your forehead. Focus on your jaw, shoulders, arms, hands, abdominal muscles, legs, and feet, in turn. Then return your focus completely to your breathing, keeping it deep and slow and even.

Many people use a sound, or mantra, during meditation in order to help retain focus. Repeating it over and over assists in clearing your head of other thoughts. The Sanskrit word "om," commonly used by Buddhists, is popular. It means "everything that ever was, is, and will be." Another helpful device is to use the word "so" on breathing in, and "hum" on breathing out.

During meditation you will find that numerous thoughts come into your mind. Don't attempt to ignore them; merely allow them to float through, as if at a distance. By consciously refocusing on your breathing, or continuously repeating a mantra, it becomes possible to limit these unwelcome intrusions, until at last they fail to register. This will not happen immediately you begin learning to meditate, but it will happen in time.

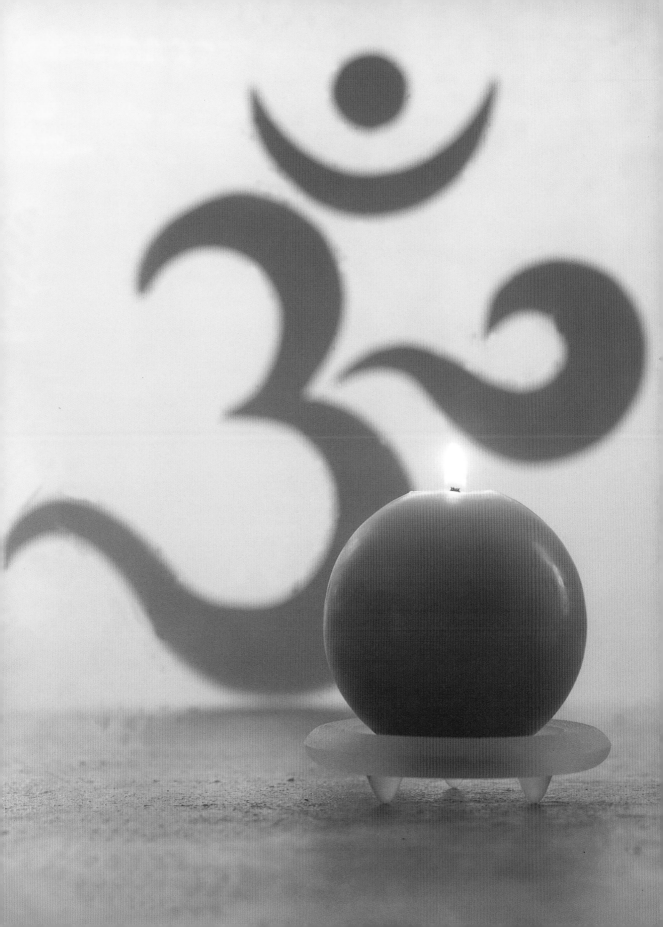

Hypnosis

There are many popular misconceptions about hypnosis, partly because it has been used for entertainment, and people think it could make them do something they don't wish to. In fact, in the hands of a skilled and qualified therapist, hypnosis utilizes a state of consciousness, somewhere between sleep and wakefulness, which is similar to daydreaming. You are not unconscious when you are hypnotized, but in a state of deep relaxation, and you continue to be fully aware of what is going on around you.

While in this trancelike state, the mind is especially receptive to positive thought. It has been said that hypnotherapy is an effective way of helping you achieve something you already want to do, whether it is giving up smoking, alleviating pain, or increasing your ability to relax and so to sleep. According to a recent study by the World Health Organization, 9 out of 10 people can be successfully hypnotized. This does not mean that you can be hypnotized against your will; in fact, the most successful hypnotherapy subjects are those who are highly motivated to make some change in their lives. People who like to stay in control of a situation, and find it difficult to trust others, are the most difficult to hypnotize.

During a hypnotic state it is possible for the therapist to help you alter the way you react to or experience a situation. For example, if the mere thought of not sleeping at night makes you anxious, and this is reinforced by actually being unable to sleep, a vicious circle develops. A hypnotherapist can help you to overcome the trigger points for insomnia that are, in effect, self-induced. If another physical or emotional problem is prohibiting sleep, and it can be helped by hypnosis, that can be the focus of treatment.

At a first consultation, the hypnotherapist will probably discuss why you think treatment could be helpful, and ask for a full history of your case, including any relevant medical or social details. The therapist should explain how he or she works, so that you know what to expect once the therapy begins. You will plan between you what you hope to achieve together. In this way, the suggestions made to you by the therapist during a session will be those that you have already agreed. The purpose of the hypnotherapy session therefore remains under your control. The first visit may involve a preliminary hypnosis session, to see how amenable you might be to treatment, before you book any subsequent session or sessions.

At the beginning of the session you will be asked to sit or lie in a comfortable position, and to try to relax. The room should be comfortable, peaceful, and conducive to relaxation. It is also essential that you feel at ease with your therapist, and able to trust him or her.

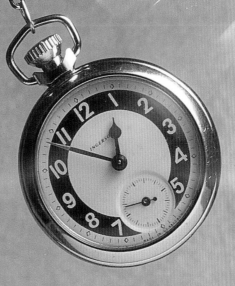

You will be guided into a trance through the gentle, repetitive words of the therapist, perhaps being encouraged to visualize a pleasant image in your mind, or to focus on a particular object in the room. Provided there is sufficient rapport between you and the therapist, this process should soon be effective. During the trance state, the therapist will talk through the issues you have previously discussed. At the end of the session, you will be gently guided out of the trance, perhaps by being told that, "When I count to five, you will wake up, feeling relaxed and refreshed, and will remember everything that has been said."

Many hypnotherapists also give their patients techniques to carry out at home, sometimes in association with a relaxation tape. Self-hypnosis can be very effective in treating sleep disorders, especially insomnia and night waking. For these problems, a series of about six sessions may be all that is needed.

▲ *Gentle repetition is a key to hypnotic technique. In the past therapists often asked clients to focus on a watch or pendant swinging on a chain. Nowadays they are more likely to ask clients to focus on a candle while they lead them into a state of hypnosis through gentle, repetitive words.*

89

Autosuggestion

Autosuggestion is a form of self-hypnosis that was developed and popularized by a French apothecary, Emile Coué, at the end of the 19th century. It is based on a form of meditation that aims to empty the mind through the repetition of positive phrases. The saying that Coué made famous was, "Every day, in every way, I am getting better and better."

▶ *Thinking positive thoughts, and being able to do this at will even when under stress, can be of enormous benefit to restful sleep.*

He believed that if a person repeated this sentence regularly at least 20 times a day, while the body was in a relaxed state, it would direct the unconscious processes of the body and mind in a positive way. This was based on the belief that the body has its own inherent ability to self-heal, and that we can promote this ability by consciously tapping into the unconscious. It is beneficial to practice relaxation and breathing exercises before embarking on a session of autosuggestion. In this way, the body and mind are more open to suggestion. Meditation can also be used in combination with autosuggestion, and a hypnotherapist may teach this technique as part of a continuing process of self-help.

Autosuggestion is frequently used to promote well-being, good health, and happiness through its emphasis on positive thought. But it can also be helpful in alleviating pain or fear, and relieving tension and anxiety. Addictions, such as smoking or drinking too much alcohol, can respond to it, and asthma and allergies may also be helped. In the case of sleep disorders, and the stress, anxiety, or fear that can contribute to them, autosuggestion has proved to be remarkably beneficial.

As with many self-help techniques, practice is imperative for autosuggestion to be effective. Once learned, however, it can be utilized at any time. Although it is perfectly possible to be entirely self-taught, the guidance and support of a teacher or therapist can be invaluable.

Coué believed that having the will to improve things was not enough if there remained a deep-seated fear that recovery was impossible. His autosuggestive techniques aimed to overcome this fear, and use the imagination in a constructive rather than a destructive way. He recommended that autosuggestion was practiced at roughly the same times each day, and under similar conditions, to benefit from the suggestibility of time and place. Whatever phrase was selected, it should be clearly positive; for example, "I am happy" is more effective than "I won't be unhappy." In the case of sleeping disorders, "I will sleep tonight" is more effective than "I won't wake up tonight."

The Silva Method

In the 1960s, a form of autosuggestion was developed in the United States by a Mexican American named José Silva. The Silva method focuses on integrating the body and mind, and uses various techniques common to cognitive therapies and autogenic training (see pages 92–93). It is sometimes described as dynamic meditation, because it works by taking the mind to a deeper, more creative level, and at this point introducing the power of positive thinking. You can follow courses with therapists trained in the Silva method, or other therapists who integrate the method into their practice.

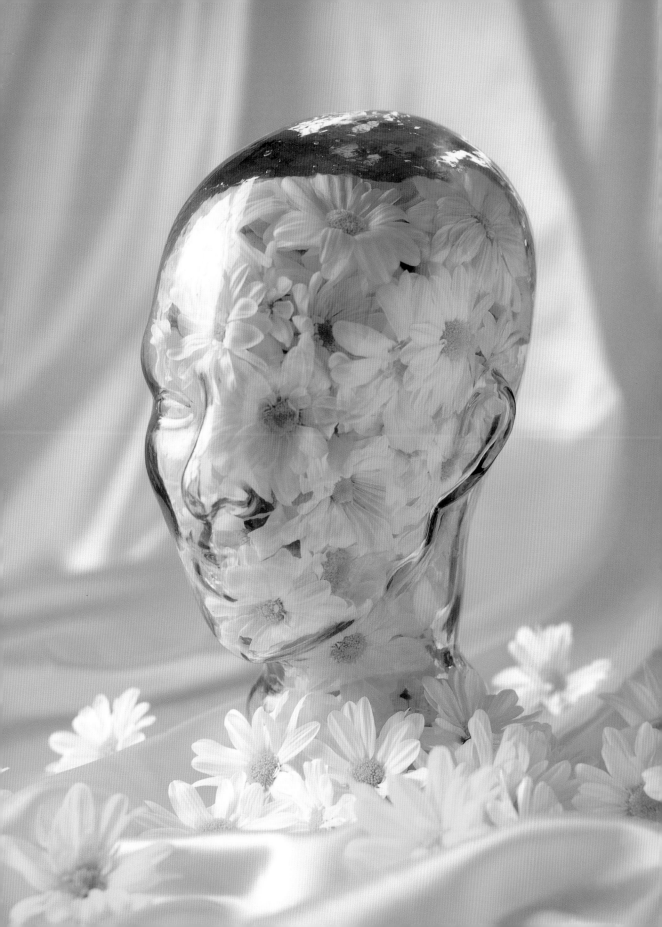

Autogenic Training

While nobody knows exactly how autogenic training works, over 300 scientific papers attest to its success in treating a variety of ailments, and improving others. These ailments include depression, colitis, high blood pressure, jet lag, migraine, and insomnia. Anyone can learn autogenic training, but it requires regular practice to be effective. Courses are taught in many hospitals and clinics, with exercises to practice at home two or three times a day. As you become more proficient, the exercises can be fitted conveniently into your daily routine.

Autogenic training was devised in the 1920s by Dr Johannes Schultz. He was already using hypnotism with many of his patients, and wondered if it would be possible to induce the same effects without hypnosis. The training is based on the principle that the body has an inherent self-healing ability, and it is possible to tap into this to affect physiological processes and treat physical illnesses. The word "autogenic" comes from the Greek, meaning self-producing.

The effects of autogenic training are both calming and invigorating. By calming the heart rate and breathing patterns, the body can make better uses of its energy resources. Many athletes and sports players find that the exercises improve their performance, and help them recover more quickly from the effects of physical exertion and injury. Autogenic training has also assisted people who want to reduce or avoid the use of sleeping pills or tranquilizers. In cases where repressed emotions, such as grief and anger, create physical discomfort and pain, autogenic training has proved effective in releasing these and providing relief.

Autogenic training requires the practice of six different exercises while in one of three positions: the reclining position, the armchair position, or the simple sitting position. The position is chosen according to circumstances. For example, the armchair position is useful for practicing while on a bus or train, or at work; the reclining position is suitable for autogenic training prior to sleep; and the simple sitting position helps to relax the neck and shoulders more fully and achieve a deeper level of relaxation. Whatever the position, you should close your eyes and focus initially on peaceful and pleasant thoughts.

While all of the exercises must be practiced in conjunction, a therapist would help a patient with a specific problem to place greater emphasis on a particular exercise. For example, the stomach exercise would be important for someone with colitis, while the heaviness and the warmth exercises would be beneficial for insomnia.

There is no doubt that the sympathetic (or autonomic) nervous system, which is mainly concerned with the workings of our internal organs, and over which we have no conscious control, responds well to autogenic training, especially when it is overactive. Another area that responds well is psychosomatic illness, in which the effects of excessive or repressed emotions are demonstrated through symptoms of physical illness. It is not surprising, therefore, that sleep disorders, which are often closely linked to our emotional well-being, are receptive to autogenic training, which reports considerable success in this area.

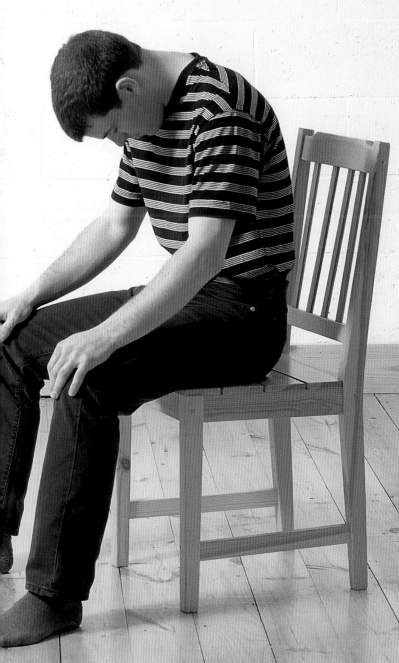

The Six Exercises

Heaviness exercise: here the focus is on feeling a heaviness in the neck, shoulders, arms, and legs. You repeat key phrases, such as "My left leg feels heavy," "My right leg feels heavy," silently again and again to induce a feeling of relaxation.

Warmth exercise: this focuses on feeling the warmth in each of the limbs, and concentrating specifically on this awareness.

Breathing exercise: focusing on breathing, increasing the depth of inhalations and slowing the speed, this increases relaxation.

Heartbeat exercise: through concentrating on the heart, in conjunction with the other exercises, it becomes possible to strengthen and calm its beat.

Stomach exercise: focusing on a feeling of warmth in the stomach and lower abdominal area helps overall relaxation, and specific relaxation of the gut.

Forehead exercise: the emphasis here is on creating a coolness of the forehead. This exercise was devised by Dr Schultz when he found that psychologically disturbed patients who were helped by taking warm baths, derived even greater relief from the application of icepacks to their foreheads.

◀ *If you practice the autogenic training exercises in the simple sitting position, you will be able to carry them out anywhere.*

Visualization

Visualization is often used in conjunction with other therapies, such as autogenic training and hypnotherapy, but it can be used effectively alone. It is more useful, however, to learn the technique from a therapist, and then practice it at home, than to be completely self-taught.

Creating images in our minds is a natural mental process – it occurs every night when we dream. This process can be used deliberately to conjure images that enhance our well-being, and that is the essence of visualization. Not only can it promote positive feelings in general, by boosting self-image, it can also support the body's ability to heal. It is thought that visualization owes its power to the close link between emotions, images, and sensations; in the same way that negative feelings, such as anger, can make you feel upset and ill, so positive feelings can have the reverse effect. Working in the United States, Dr Carl Simonton pioneered the use of visualization with cancer patients. The technique involved creating mental images of healthy body cells attacking and destroying cancer cells.

For sufferers from sleep disorders and insomnia, visualization can be an effective method of emptying the mind of troubled, distressing, or overstimulating images. It is also thought to be beneficial in stress reduction and relaxation, which makes it an additional aid to sleep. Thinking in images, which uses the right side of the brain, is believed to be helpful in balancing the activity of the overused left side of the brain. Integrating the more creative and intuitive aspect of the right side of the brain may help to achieve a beneficial mental balance.

Before beginning visualization, do at least five minutes of relaxation and breathing exercises (see pages 83 and 85). When your mind and body are in a relaxed state, consciously imagine some peaceful place. Notice as many details as you can: the quality of the light, the temperature, the smell, the form of your surroundings, whether natural or manmade – the sensation of the ground underfoot, for example. The image should be apprehended in as sensuous a way as possible: use your imagination to make you aware of all the sights and sensations of the scene that you are visualizing.

At first, it can be difficult to conjure up an image from nowhere, especially if you are not a particularly visual person. Find a picture in a book, or a photograph of a vacation spot that holds happy memories, and study it closely, using it as a cue to other, non-visual feelings. Look at it for several minutes, then close your eyes, and picture it in your mind, visualizing the details. Recreate it as fully as you can, with all of the little elements that will bring it to life.

This process can be hard initially, which is why it can be useful to have a therapist to guide you through it. With practice, however, it becomes much easier. If you want to achieve a state of peaceful sleepiness, it won't be long before calling up a particular image, and then taking a short journey through that image, will open the way to repose.

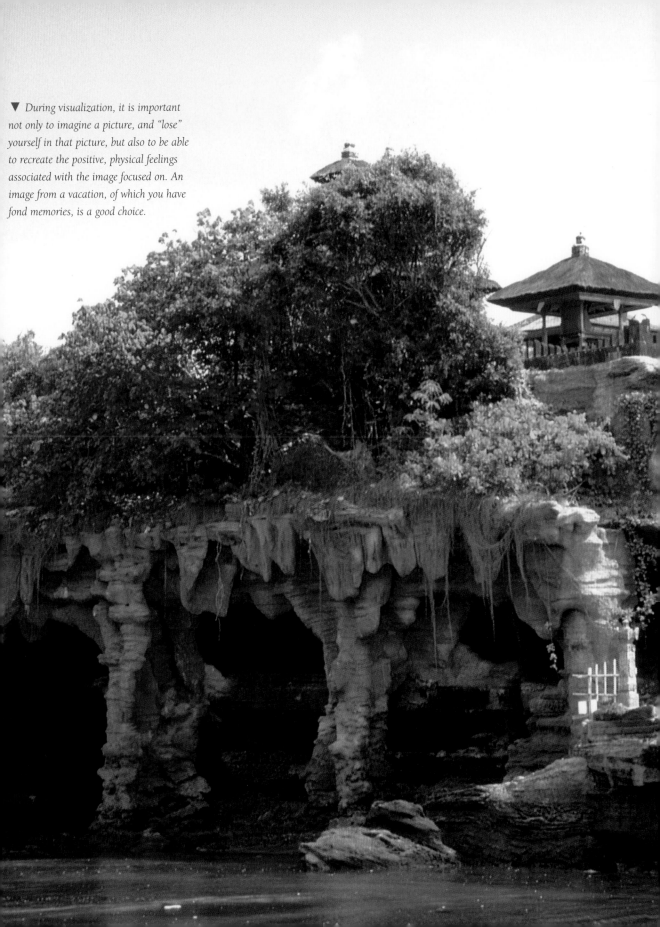

▼ During visualization, it is important not only to imagine a picture, and "lose" yourself in that picture, but also to be able to recreate the positive, physical feelings associated with the image focused on. An image from a vacation, of which you have fond memories, is a good choice.

Acupuncture and Acupressure

Traditional Chinese medicine is based on the premise that the body's energy (*qi*) runs along invisible pathways (meridians), and that if these pathways become blocked, the resulting imbalance can cause illness. Acupoints occur along the meridians, and by stimulating or relaxing these – with a needle in acupuncture or with pressure in acupressure – energy can be released and the body can begin to heal itself. The Japanese equivalent of acupressure, based on the same principles, is known as shiatsu.

The traditional Chinese diagnosis of disorders and illnesses is more subtle than the orthodox Western approach. It is also more holistic. For example, the cause of insomnia may be that the kidneys are not receiving enough cool and relaxing energy, because the meridians are blocked. One way of relieving this disorder is to practice the deep, diaphragmatic breathing techniques described on page 85, in conjunction with the treatment of the acupressure point kidney 6. Acupuncture and acupressure can be used to boost the body's energy, or to disperse energy blockages, according to need. Practitioners also aim to balance the *yin* and *yang* energies of the body: *yin* and *yang* are represented as cold and hot; female and male; expansive, relaxing and energetic, and inward-looking, earthy, and fiery. Illness is thought to occur if the two forces are stagnant, or out of balance. Acupuncture must always be carried out by a qualified practitioner, but acupressure can easily be done at home – although it is wise to take expert advice initially to gain full benefit.

A number of acupressure points are indicated for treating insomnia. These include gall bladder 12, which is situated two fingers' width behind the ear, where there is a small indentation under the bone of the skull. Heart governor 8 is located in the center of the palm of the hand. Find this point by bending the middle finger to touch the palm, then press upward into the hand, toward the base of the middle finger. Once located, apply pressure to the point with the index finger of your other hand. CV 17, also helpful for insomnia, is found in the center of the chest.

Acupuncture and acupressure can also treat the disorders of which insomnia or sleep disturbances may be a symptom. Anxiety, stress, and tension can respond well: so can chronic pain, which may contribute to a sleep problem. Massaging acupoint heart 7, on the inside of the wrist, in line with the little finger, can steady heart palpitations, and has a generally sedating effect. Pericardium 6, situated three fingers' width down from the wrist between the tendons of the arm, and usually recommended for nausea and sickness, helps to stop the mind racing and to control panicky thoughts, which can help aid sleep. Governing vessel 26, located just below the nose, in the groove of the upper lip, is the acupoint recommended for the relief of depression, which may contribute to early morning waking. This point, however, should not be stimulated for longer than one minute, and pressure must be light, since it can raise blood pressure. It should only be used for short periods.

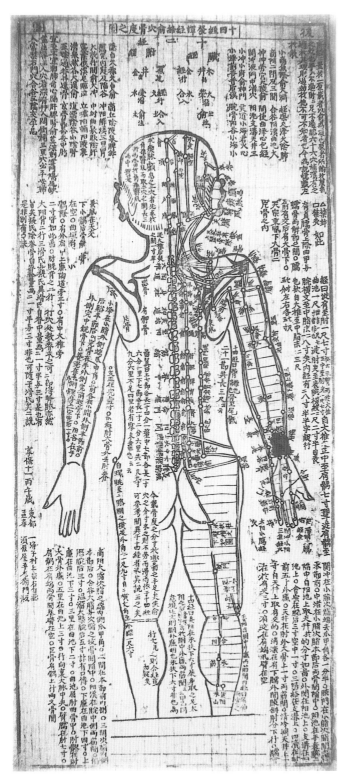

▼ *Acupressure can be applied to points situated along the energy meridians running through the body to promote relaxation and aid sleep. Heart 7 (below) has a sedating effect; pericardium 6 (center) stops persistent, panicky thoughts and calms the mind; kidney 6 (bottom) can treat insomnia by promoting relaxation.*

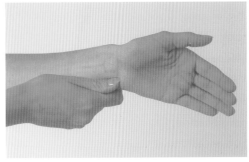

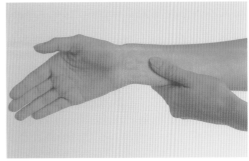

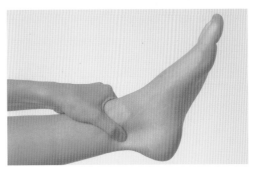

◄ *The energy pathways, or meridians, used by practitioners today have been in existence and used successfully in acupuncture, acupressure, and shiatsu for thousands of years. The meridian chart featured here originates from 19th-century Japan.*

Reflexology

Reflexology is sometimes referred to as "zone therapy," because it relies on the principle that the body can be divided into zones, and that applying pressure to one area of a zone affects the energy flow in another part of the same zone. This approach makes it possible to treat inaccessible disorders – such as headaches and migraines, for example – by applying pressure elsewhere within the same zone. Treatment is usually administered to reflex points in the feet, but occasionally in the hands, that correspond to areas or organs of the body sharing the same energy lines within the same zones.

▶ *A foot massage is extremely relaxing. Reflexologists believe that areas of the feet correspond to parts of the body, and that by manipulating a specific "zone" on the feet, the corresponding area of the body will also be treated. Sessions with a qualified therapist will bring greatest benefit, but you can also learn how to do it for yourself.*

Reflexology is an ancient therapy, thought to have developed in China, alongside acupuncture, over 4500 years ago. There is also evidence of its use in ancient Egypt, from wall paintings in the physician's tomb at Saqqara, dating from 2330 BC. It is often utilized as part of a combined approach to a problem, alleviating contributory factors or specific ailments. It can enhance the effects of a generalized massage, for example, or act as a self-help practice to promote relaxation and sleep before going to bed.

Reflexology is also used to diagnose the causes of problems. For example, if night waking results from sweating linked to the hormonal changes of the menopause, reflexology would determine and treat the imbalance. A skilled practitioner can "read" the feet, feeling any crystallized deposits that might reflect blockages and tensions in the energy flow. These can then be gently stimulated and dispersed.

Reflexology can be an effective self-help therapy for an acute or chronic sleep problem, but it is useful to consult a trained reflexologist for initial advice and treatment. The holistic approach ensures that any therapy is individually prescribed, and takes into account all aspects of your physical and mental well-being. You can be shown reflexology points to use as a self-help measure and as part of an overall, personalized approach to your problem.

A general foot massage can soothe the system, as well as being a very pleasant experience. But reflexology also treats specific symptoms that can disrupt sleep. Incontinence and bedwetting can be treated by massaging the reflex points corresponding to the kidneys, adrenals, bladder muscles, and prostate. Stress can be alleviated by massaging the reflexes for the solar plexus, head, and heart. Muscle tension causing pain in the neck and shoulders can be eased by massaging reflex points in the area below the toes.

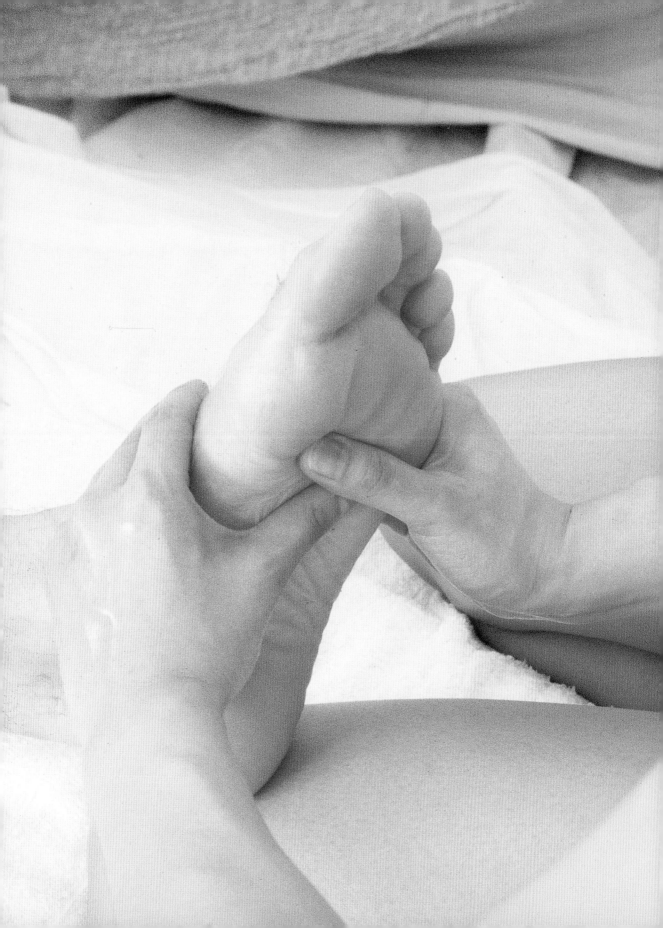

Osteopathy

Osteopathy focuses on the mechanics of the body, and can both diagnose and treat problems. It is an holistic approach to the musculo-skeletal system – the spine, joints, muscles, connective tissue, and ligaments – based on the principle that if this system is out of alignment, it can affect the working of the entire body.

Osteopathy can treat the musculo-skeletal pain that disturbs sleep. Back and neck pain is particularly responsive, and so is osteoarthritis – but not rheumatoid arthritis, which is an inflammatory disease. Symptoms of asthma, constipation, and menstrual pain can also be alleviated by osteopathy. Treatment must be given by a qualified practitioner, and symptoms are normally relieved in three to six sessions of 30–45 minutes each.

Osteopathic techniques are varied, and are not limited to the high-velocity thrusts that give osteopaths the reputation for "cracking" bones when releasing the muscular tension between two vertebrae, for example. The noise is actually caused by air bubbles, located in the synovial (lubricating) fluid of the joints, which pop under the pressure of the movements. Osteopaths also use massage techniques to loosen stiff muscles; articulatory techniques – in which a limb is supported through a range of movements to provide passive stretching of ligaments – to restore joint mobility; and friction to improve blood circulation to an area.

In addition to its direct effects, osteopathy can have a more subtle influence on different internal organs and activities of the body. Relieving musculo-skeletal stress can affect deeper levels, removing the tension that might be causing underactivity within a particular organ or gland. This has proved to be the case in some hormonal problems, for example, where secretions from an endocrine gland are improved through osteopathy. In insomnia, this might have implications in the secretion of melatonin from the pineal gland in the brain.

▶ *Even in adult life, the possibility of minute movement between the joints of the skull bones still exist. This is exploited in cranial osteopathy to help relieve tension in the flow of cerebro-spinal fluid.*

Cranial Osteopathy

This requires additional, specialized osteopathic training, because here the practitioner focuses on the skull, vertebral column, and pelvic area, and the effects of any misalignment on the flow of cerebrospinal fluid within them. The brain and parts of the nervous system are bathed in cerebro-spinal fluid, which needs to flow freely for the nervous system to work to its best advantage. Tensions can result in blockages that provoke a variety of physical symptoms, including headaches and migraine, sight problems, and stress disorders. Cranial osteopathy must be carried out by a qualified practitioner, who will often utilize a full range of osteopathy techniques.

Chiropractic

This is a development of osteopathy, formulated by Canadian osteopath David Daniel Palmer, working in the late 1800s. The focus of treatment is the spine, based on the principle that the swift but gentle realignment of the vertebrae relieves pain in the immediate area of the back. It can also alleviate irritable bowel syndrome, period problems, and asthma in some patients, which can be termed an indirect result of treatment. It is most likely to be helpful in sleep difficulties caused by back pain, or discomfort associated with postural problems.

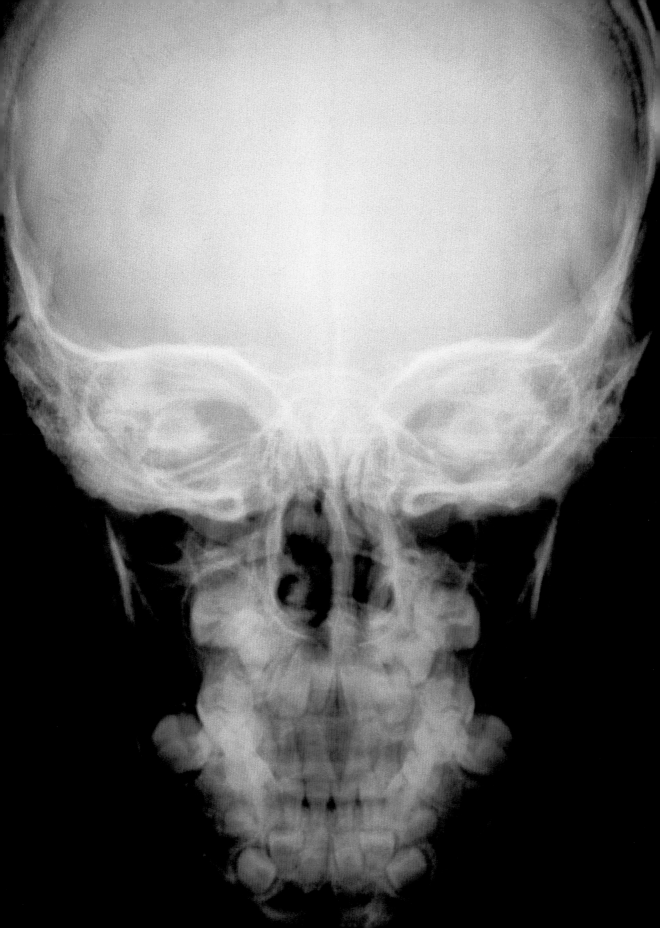

Herbal Remedies

A number of herbal remedies can be extremely effective for sleep disorders, and they are recommended for both acute and chronic symptoms of insomnia. Many herbal remedies are available over-the-counter from drugstores, pharmacies, and health food stores, and herbal teas can often be found in local supermarkets.

A qualified medical herbalist prescribes according to specific symptoms, taking an holistic approach to the individual. Treatment may be given in the form of whole plants which need making up into a decoction, tincture, or tea. There are also many over-the-counter remedies available. If these prove ineffective, it is still worth consulting a herbal practitioner, who has a range of around 200 plants to choose from in prescribing treatment.

Herbal medicines are derived from the entire plant, unlike pharmaceutical medicines that are produced by synthesizing the active component of the plant in the laboratory. Herbal medicines can have a potent effect, and need to be treated with respect. Many conditions respond favorably to them – including stress-related disorders, skin complaints, menstrual problems, high blood pressure, stomach ulcers, headaches, arthritis, and colds.

One of the most effective natural tranquilizers is valerian, which is often found in herbal remedies prescribed for insomnia. The root of the plant has the greatest potency, and it has been used regularly from the mid-16th century to treat nervous disorders such as epilepsy, anxiety, and insomnia. Numerous studies have indicated the effectiveness of valerian, and research carried out in Switzerland by Leathwood and Chauffard in 1985 concluded that valerian was "active early in the night, that it improved sleep quality, and produced no hangover after-effects the next day."

Passionflower (*Passiflora*) is often prescribed by herbalists for recurrent insomnia, anxiety, and tension. Herbalists use this singly, or in combination with other herbs, according to the individual's needs. Hops, the chief constituent of beer, are a valuable source of natural tranquilizing properties, but only in their original form – drinking large quantities of beer will exacerbate, not cure, sleep disorders. Some of the many other herbs that are valued for their relaxing and anxiety-reducing properties are chamomile, lemon balm, wild lettuce, lime tree flowers, motherwort, and Californian poppy.

Herbal remedies can, of course, also treat any underlying illnesses that contribute to sleep disorders. A herb considered effective for depression – particularly when associated with the menopause – is St John's Wort (*Hypericum*). It is often used by herbal therapists for sleep remedies where depression is a significant feature.

Herbal Pillows

A herbal pillow may help to induce sleep, especially as you begin to associate its fragrance with bedtime. Buy a ready-made pillow, or make your own, using a fine-grain strong white cotton cloth for the internal pillowcase and stuffing it with herbs such as dried lavender, hops, and chamomile. Choose from the scents you particularly like, and bear in mind that dried herbs will eventually lose their fragrance and need replacing.

Cautions

Herbal medicines are extremely potent, so it is essential to follow all instructions carefully, and to observe the following precautions:

- Never exceed the stated dose.
- Do not use herbal remedies if you are pregnant or breastfeeding unless advised by a qualified practitioner.
- Do not take herbal remedies for prolonged periods of time.
- Stop using a remedy immediately if you experience any side-effects.
- Do not collect herbs from the wild.
- Only buy over-the-counter remedies if the packet states what it contains.
- Always advise any herbalist you consult about other drugs you are taking.

◀ *Making a herbal pillow is quite simple. Remember to replace the dried herbs after about 9–12 months.*

Homeopathy

Homeopathy is based on the principle that "like cures like." This means that a little of what causes a problem will also stimulate the body to heal itself, and homeopathy uses tiny amounts of its chosen substances, heavily diluted. The greater the dilution, the greater the potency of the remedy – the reverse of the way in which orthodox medicines usually work. Remedies come in strengths of ×6, ×12, ×30, and ×100.

Homeopathy was established in the late 18th century by a medically trained German doctor, Samuel Hahnemann. While conducting experiments on himself, Hahnemann discovered that quinine produced the symptoms of malaria – the disease that it is used to alleviate. From his research, he formulated the three main principles on which homeopathy is based.

• A substance that produces a set of symptoms in a healthy person can be used to cure the same symptoms in someone who is sick.

• Continued dilution of a substance increases its potency and its ability to cure symptoms, without producing unwanted side-effects.

• Homeopathy is a holistic treatment, and takes into account the patient's emotional as well as physical symptoms.

Homeopathy was used extensively by the London Homeopathic Hospital during the cholera epidemic of 1854, when their cure rate was 60 percent, compared with 16 percent of the general population. It is an increasingly popular therapy, which counts Queen Elizabeth and other members of the British royal family among its users.

Homeopathy can be effective in treating disorders that give rise to poor sleep and sleep problems themselves. Because of the therapy's holistic nature, it is advisable to consult an experienced and qualified homeopathic practitioner – it takes skill to match the right remedy to the presenting symptoms. However, homeopathic remedies are widely available over-the-counter, and you can diagnose and treat yourself. Bear in mind the following points when taking remedies, to help them work more effectively.

• Remedies come in a variety of forms: granules, powders, tablets, pills, and drops. Handle them as little as possible, and place them in a clean spoon before putting them in your mouth.

• Only the person taking the remedy should touch it, so as not to contaminate it and reduce its efficacy.

• Keep the remedies away from strong and pungent substances that could destroy their benefits: peppermint, eucalyptus, and coffee, for example.

• Do not clean your teeth, drink tea or coffee, or eat anything just prior to taking a remedy. Rinse your mouth with clean water and wait five minutes if you are not sure.

▶ *More and more people are now using homeopathy to treat a wide range of physical complaints and illnesses, including sleep disorders. Place the remedy on a clean spoon before putting it in your mouth.*

Homeopathic Remedies

Below are some remedies especially recommended for insomnia and other sleep problems.

Symptoms	Remedy
Insomnia and fear that sleep will never come again	Ignatia
Insomnia with fear caused by fright	Aconite
Insomnia with irritability	Nux vomica

Take the above remedies in ×30 strength, one pill each night, one hour before bed, for 10 nights. The remedy can be taken again on waking in the night, if necessary. Do not exceed the recommended dose, since the remedy may "prove" and become ineffective.

Remedies recommended for snoring are either aconite ×30, one pill at bedtime for 10 nights, or natrum muriaticum, in the same dose. Other homeopathic remedies are suitable for problems implicated in sleep disorders: for example, ignatia or pulsatilla for depression; and arsenicum albicans for anxiety combined with restlessness. However, many problems associated with sleep disturbance are emotional, and in that case a consultation will be useful in determining a remedy that considers the origins as well as their symptomatic effect.

Bach Flower Remedies

British homeopath Dr Edward Bach spent 20 years in the early part of this century researching the effects of personality and mental outlook on disease, and developing the use of flower remedies. His therapy has been popular ever since. There are 38 flower remedies, distilled from the essence of flower petals, and usually preserved in alcohol, although this is not essential.

▶ *Flower remedies are best taken directly onto the tongue from a dropper. Rinsing the mouth with clean water is necessary before taking them, to avoid contamination – from coffee, for example.*

Remedies are stored in little bottles, and dispensed directly onto the tongue, through a dropper: only two to three drops are needed at a time. Dr Bach, who had trained as a physician and bacteriologist, believed that the body had its own self-healing ability, but this could become blocked by long-standing worries or fears, which hindered recovery. Flower remedies are thought to help a person regain psychological peace, allowing the body's energies to flow freely again, and any necessary healing to be completed. So flower remedies have no direct effect on physical symptoms, but on the mind's ability to influence the body's response to these.

The Bach Rescue Remedy – a combination of five flower remedies designed to deal with everyday emergencies – contains clematis, impatiens, rock rose, cherry plum, and star of Bethlehem. It is additional to the 38 regular remedies, and is thought to help prevent snoring problems. But flower remedies can be most useful in treating the emotional factors that can give rise to sleep problems, whether these are recurrent or once-only difficulties. Flower remedies can be used singly or in combination with one another; their aim is to counteract negative states of mind. Bach flower remedies can be especially useful in conjunction with other therapies, such as meditation and autosuggestion. They can also be valuable in acute situations, where you know that feelings of stress, tension, and even jet lag could benefit from a helping hand.

Flower Remedies for Sleep Disorders

Agrimony	Hiding worries behind a brave façade	**Rock rose**	Alarmed, panicky
Aspen	Apprehensive but for no known reason	**Star of Bethlehem**	Fright, after-effects of bad news
Cherry plum	Uncontrollable, irrational thoughts	**Sweet chestnut**	Despair, dejected thoughts, and bleak outlook
Elm	Overwhelmed by responsibility	**Walnut**	Adjustment to transition or change, e.g. moving home, divorce, menopause
Gentian	Despondency		
Holly	Jealousy and suspicion		
Impatiens	Irritability and impatience	**White chestnut**	Persistent unwanted thoughts and worries
Larch	Fear of failure	**Willow**	Resentment
Red chestnut	Obsessed by concern for others		

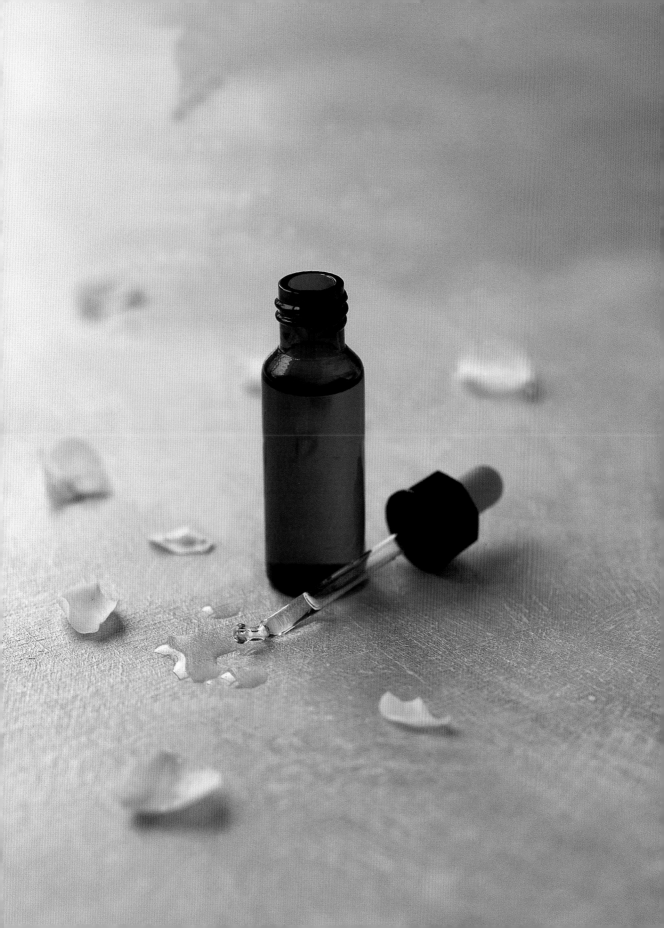

Feng Shui

Like all Eastern medicine and philosophies, the principles of feng shui (pronounced *foong shway*) are based on an understanding of the subtle movement of an electromagnetic flow of energy. This energy is referred to as *qi* or *chi* in China and Japan, and *prana* in India. It is thought to flow within the body along meridians – invisible pathways that are utilized in acupuncture, acupressure, and shiatsu – and to be concentrated in certain areas of the body.

Qi is believed to be either *yin* or *yang*, the opposite and complementary energies which must be balanced to enable the body and mind to work at their best. Thoughts, emotions, and feelings can affect our *qi* energy, and our level of *qi* can affect how we feel emotionally. In addition to our inner energy, *qi* is thought to extend from 4 to 40in (10 to 100cm) beyond the body, and to exist within the world around us, so that it can be affected by the space in which it is confined. Feng shui is a way of understanding, and working with, the movement of energy within a certain space. Its effects are claimed to benefit not only health, well-being, and relationships, but even such material matters as financial income and material success.

Although it is a complex and subtle approach to the use of natural energies both within and outside us, some principles of feng shui can be adapted to good effect. One area where feng shui can be especially useful is in the bedroom, where it can be helpful in tackling sleep problems. Keep sharp and shiny furniture with metallic reflective surfaces out of the bedroom. It increases *yang* energy, which tends to make the atmosphere more aggressive and tensed, ready for action and not conducive to sleep. Objects that promote calmer and more relaxing *yin* energy are natural in origin: wooden furniture with rounded corners, natural fabrics, neutral and soothing colors, plants with rounded, floppy leaves. If the room is rectangular, positioning of furniture and other objects is fairly easy, but if it is L-shaped, or there are additional angular features, these need to be softened to avoid *qi* swirling too fast at these points. Mirrors, which reflect *qi* back, should not be placed opposite the bed, because the reflecting activity will be too stimulating. Move them, or cover them at night to avoid this problem.

The direction in which the room, and more importantly the bed, faces also affects *qi*, and how it flows through the body during sleep. If you find the ideal location for your bed, time spent asleep should optimize the flow of *qi*, so that you awake each morning feeling refreshed. The first consideration is whether your bed faces north, south, east, or west. Use a compass to figure this out. The direction in which the top of your head points is the most important.

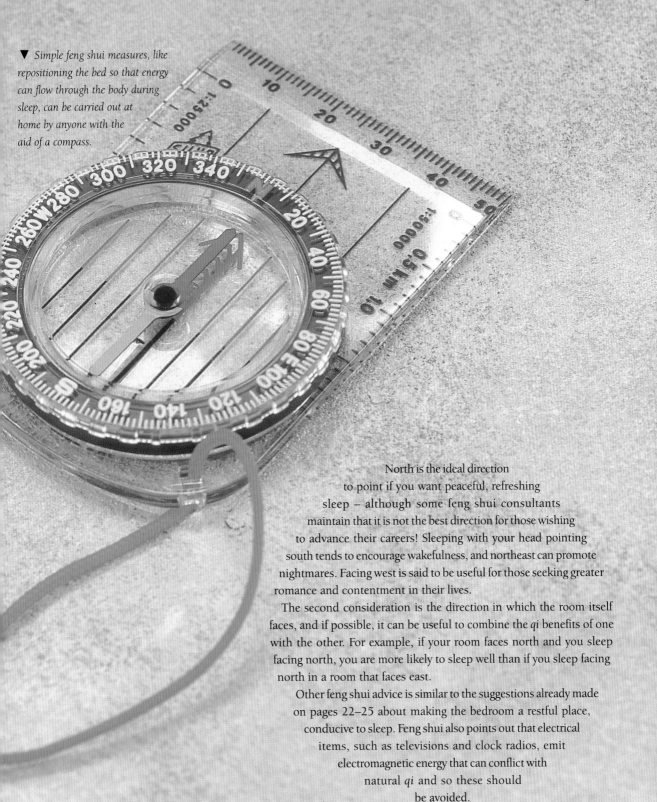

▼ *Simple feng shui measures, like repositioning the bed so that energy can flow through the body during sleep, can be carried out at home by anyone with the aid of a compass.*

North is the ideal direction to point if you want peaceful, refreshing sleep – although some feng shui consultants maintain that it is not the best direction for those wishing to advance their careers! Sleeping with your head pointing south tends to encourage wakefulness, and northeast can promote nightmares. Facing west is said to be useful for those seeking greater romance and contentment in their lives.

The second consideration is the direction in which the room itself faces, and if possible, it can be useful to combine the *qi* benefits of one with the other. For example, if your room faces north and you sleep facing north, you are more likely to sleep well than if you sleep facing north in a room that faces east.

Other feng shui advice is similar to the suggestions already made on pages 22–25 about making the bedroom a restful place, conducive to sleep. Feng shui also points out that electrical items, such as televisions and clock radios, emit electromagnetic energy that can conflict with natural *qi* and so these should be avoided.

Index

Credits

Quarto would like to acknowledge and thank the following for providing pictures used in this book.

Dunlopillo UK: page 7 (below); e.t. archive: page 9 (above); Image Bank: pages 6, 7 (above), 8 (below) and 67 (above); Michelle Pickering: page 13 (top); Pictor: page 101; Tony Stone: page 8 (above).

All other photographs are the copyright of Quarto.

Quarto would also like to thank Mark Jenkins for his help in the making of this publication. Mark is a London-based composer of film, theater, and commercial music, who has several albums available worldwide on the AMP Records label.

AMP Records
Box 387, London N22 6SF, UK
Tel/Fax: +44 (0)181 889 0616
World Wide Web: http://www.ampmusic.demon.co.uk
E-mail: info@ampmusic.demon.co.uk

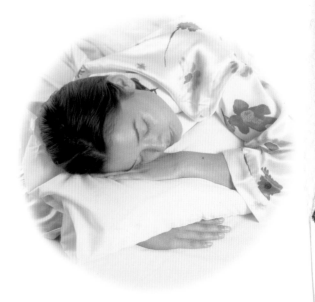